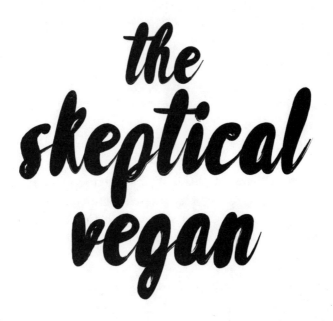

the skeptical vegan

my journey from notorious meat eater to tofu-munching vegan —a survival guide

eric c. lindstrom

Foreword by Victoria Moran

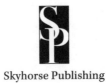

Skyhorse Publishing

Skyhorse Publishing books may be purchased in bulk at special discounts for sales promotion, corporate gifts, fund-raising, or educational purposes. Special editions can also be created to specifications. For details, contact the Special Sales Department, Skyhorse Publishing, 307 West 36th Street, 11th Floor, New York, NY 10018 or info@ skyhorsepublishing.com.

Skyhorse® and Skyhorse Publishing® are registered trademarks of Skyhorse Publishing, Inc.®, a Delaware corporation.

Visit our website at www.skyhorsepublishing.com.

10 9 8 7 6 5 4 3 2 1

Library of Congress Cataloging-in-Publication Data is available on file.

Cover design by Eric C. Lindstrom
Cover photo credit: Eric C. Lindstrom

Print ISBN: 978-1-5107-1760-2
Ebook ISBN: 978-1-5107-1761-9

Printed in the United States of America

This book is dedicated to
Jen, my vegan wife;
our vegan babies;
and our vegan dog.

TABLE OF CONTENTS

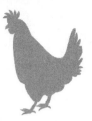

FOREWORD

I am fascinated by the relatively rare and uniquely human phenomenon of transformation. The best stories are those that tell of overcoming, redemption, and glorious *afters* contrasting with prosaic *befores*. *The Skeptical Vegan* is a story like that: relevant, inspiring, instructive, and laugh-out-loud funny.

Eric Lindstrom isn't just a skeptical vegan; he's an honest one. He shares every pitfall, inconvenience, and temptation of this journey, while at the same time tempting us with its possibilities: physical renewal, a genuinely sustainable way to live on planet earth, and the ability to look at a cow or pig or chicken without the subconscious guilt of a predator who was never meant to be one.

I relate to Eric's experiences on many levels. Like him, I approached veganism obese and ravenous. Food was my drug, and only rich foods—meat, cheese, ice cream, pastries—counted. Fruits and vegetables were garnishes, and grains a mere foil for butter and Alfredo sauce.

While Eric's original impetus for going vegan was a bet with his wife he couldn't bear to lose, I wanted to take this step for the animals. I knew that vast numbers of them were, and are, abused and slaughtered in an agricultural system confidently assuring us that their sacrificed bodies are "what's for dinner." My spirit was all in, but my flesh weakened in the face of a fluffy cheddar omelet or carrot cake with cream cheese frosting.

The details of my turnaround are different from Eric's, as yours are or will be, but the result is the same: a way of eating that offers health (for me, that includes over sixty pounds left behind decades ago) and a way of living that promises purpose. The choice I've made, as well as Eric and other vegans, combined with a significant reduction in animal food consumption by millions more, means that we're killing half a billion fewer animals in the US annually than we were ten years ago. We did that. And we can do more.

My only complaint about the book you're now holding is that it ends. That's okay, though, because when it's over you get to have your own adventures. And as you create your vegan story, you can carry with you the thought: "If that guy could do this—good Lord, he practically ate entire carcasses! —I can do it for sure." A better life awaits, and a kinder, saner world—but first: a really good read.

Victoria Moran
Author, *Main Street Vegan*
Host, Main Street Vegan podcast
Director, Main Street Vegan Academy

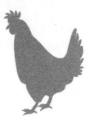

INTRODUCTION

We strive for a world where every earthling has the right to live and grow.
That's why we don't eat animals.
—Ruby Roth

This book is a love story. About a man and his meat. A love that couldn't last forever.

We live in a world where 97 percent of the population considers that animals are food. That somehow, opposable thumbs rocketed us to the top of the food chain. This perceived superiority is evidenced nightly on our dinner plates, which traditionally are centered around meat. Mammals, birds, fish, even reptiles. No meal is complete without some form of meat drowning in some amount of brown gravy.

I know this as a fact, since I lived this way for the first half of my life. I was a notorious, unstoppable, insatiable meat eater for the "better" part of my life.

And then one day, I woke up. Vegan.

This book is meant to inspire. Like the 1980 United States men's Olympic hockey team. But replace the hockey puck with a millet patty, the hockey sticks with carrot sticks, and the Russians with bacon. No one ever imagined that the meat could be beat. It was a true "Miracle on Rice."

My story proves that anyone can turn their lives around and go vegan. For their own health, for the environment, *and* for the animals. Whether you're currently a vegetarian so addicted to cheese you're unable to take that next step or a full-on meat eater who might be curious about what it would take to lead a healthier vegan lifestyle, this book details the drama of my own personal journey from carnivore to skeptical herbivore and, eventually, on to ethical vegan. It proves that anyone, *at any age*, can become a card-carrying, tofu-loving, hemp milk-drinking vegan. *Even if* they currently start every day with over easy eggs, crispy bacon, buttered toast, Greek yogurt, and cream in their coffee.

To say I had a penchant for meat is an understatement. Imagine, for a moment, William Shakespeare's *Romeo and Juliet*. But I'm Romeo, and Juliet is meat. I stand below meat's balcony, the moonlight glistening off her fat. But, soft! What light through yonder window breaks?

"Good night, good night! Parting is such sweet sorrow, that I shall say goodnight till it bone marrow," Juliet says. "What's in a name? That which we call a roast. By any other name would smell as sweet."

Or taste as sweet. I can't lie: a roast tasted sweet. I was madly in love with meat.

Growing up, I only read Dr. Seuss's *Green Eggs and Ham*. As a teenager, I listened to nothing but Meatloaf. Later in life, Kevin Bacon was my favorite actor and *Meatballs* was my favorite movie. I pretty much ate meat, or some animal-derived food, with every meal.

It took me more than forty years to finally turn my life around in more ways than one by becoming vegan—overnight. Went to bed masticating meat, woke up pigging out on plants.

Throughout this book, you'll find out why being vegan is a *lifestyle* and not a *diet*, and that there are varying levels of veganism, from Level 0 to Level 11. A sliding scale challenges the notion of a dichotomy that says, technically, you're either a vegan or you're not. More on this later. Of course, the notion of rating anyone based on a number is completely wrong and ridiculous. But, for the record, I'm a solid Vegan Level 8.

The bottom-line definition all vegans agree on when it comes to a vegan diet is that we don't consume meat, fish and seafood, dairy, or eggs. Meat includes all marine life, and dairy includes butter, cheese, yogurt, and ice cream—in case you were going to ask. In addition to this *dietary* guideline, vegans try to live their lives with as little impact on the planet, the environment, and animals as possible by not supporting overtly nonvegan companies. This is outwardly represented by not wearing or using leather, wool, or silk (or any other material derived from an animal) and by purchasing toiletries and other household items that are "certified vegan" and "cruelty-free." Keep in mind that some cosmetics may be labeled "cruelty-free" and still contain animal ingredients. I know, it's a lot to keep track of.

It's not always easy to do, but it's always easy to try.

You will sometimes hear people refer to a "whole-food, plant-based diet" (WFPB), which might be confusing, since it sounds like it requires shopping at Whole Foods, which sells *a lot* of meat. A WFPB has nothing to do with the grocery store chain. It's a way of eating healthy. Some vegans eat a WFPB, but some people who eat a WFPB for their health are not vegan. There are millions of people who subscribe to a whole-food, plant-based diet and who still may support animal testing or wear assless leather chaps, for example. And it should be noted: all chaps are assless.

These same plant-based individuals oftentimes refer to themselves as "vegan," in the interest of a catchier moniker that others would understand, evidenced on the majority of "vegan" food packaging, but these individuals aren't *ethically* vegan.

Vegans live by *ahimsa*—in the Hindu, Buddhist, and Jain traditions—a word in Sanskrit that means "do no harm" and is the principle of nonviolence toward *all* living things. Vegans escort spiders out of their bathrooms and will actually risk their own lives by pulling the car over on a busy highway to help a wounded turtle in the middle of the road. Really. I know a vegan who did that.

To review: vegans eat plant-based diets and *also* do everything they can, every day of their lives, to not bring additional, unnecessary harm onto the planet, others, or animals. Individuals on a plant-based diet benefit from the incredible health advantages of eating fruits, vegetables, and whole grains, but they may not truly make "the ethical connection."

Throughout this book, I'll use the word *vegan* in both the dietary and ethical senses but will highlight the notable differences between vegan and plant-based as needed. An excellent example of this distinction is Dr. T. Colin Campbell, one of the world's leading authorities on plant-based nutrition, who doesn't consider himself vegan.

Conversely, vegans may not always eat the healthiest diets but will eventually, probably, lose weight and feel great by eliminating meat, dairy, and eggs—unless they eat a vegan diet of nothing but potato chips and root beer. Seriously, though, most vegans who start out doing it for ethical reasons end up on the health track, too. In fact, some people feel that a vegan diet is the easiest way to get your health back on track because there are so many incredible food options that will accidently make you healthier.

I didn't change, I just woke up.
—Anonymous

This book will take you through my own trials and tribulations of becoming vegan and includes everything from living a happy and healthy life without meat to giving up cheese and eggs to replacing your leather jacket and shoes to assimilating yourself at a vegan potluck. If you follow along and have the will to change, you can easily transition to veganism overnight—like I did. Or, maybe you will take a week or two. Or even a month. The point is, with this book in hand, you'll know that it *is* possible and that there are incredible benefits to becoming vegan.

Vegans are a mysterious breed. Under normal conditions, one can't easily spot a vegan in the wild, but there are some important tips that will make living your life as a vegan more pleasurable. If you're ever curious if a person standing next to you at the local pub might be vegan, the easiest way to tell is to offer them something to eat—even a vegetable. When approached with food, a vegan will immediately let you know they're vegan. Even if that food *is* vegan. In fact, just by approaching a vegan and starting a conversation about anything, they will begin to shake . . . holding back with all their might . . . prepared to strike at any moment . . . poised . . . ready to let you know: They. Are. Vegan.

In order for you to fully understand, appreciate, and peacefully live among modern vegans, published here for the first time anywhere is my exclusive "Know Your Vegan" checklist. Like a ten-point auto inspection, this list tells you what to look for when trying to spot a vegan in the wild.

Vegans will inevitably let you know they are vegan. As I said, we can't help it. Any conversation will lead to this, so be prepared with a response. Something along the lines of "Oh, that's nice" will do. Never ask, "Why?" Or, "Would you eat an animal if you were stranded on a desert island and were otherwise going to die?" Or, "Where do you get your protein?" These questions may force the vegan to strike. Possibly throw a vegan Birkenstock at you. Or maybe just throw a fit. You'll craft your own responses to all these questions, and countless more, over time as you transition to veganism. An excellent resource for all answers vegan is the book *Mind If I Order the Cheeseburger?: And Other Questions People Ask Vegans* by Sherry Colb, Cornell Law Professor, ethical vegan, contributor to this book, and someone I am honored to call my friend.

Vegans will educate themselves. They are fully prepared to answer any questions about anything vegan. And healthy living. And pretty much any other subject. Go ahead, ask them what's so bad about honey . . . or silk. They have an answer. They've watched *Forks Over Knives* and *Cowspiracy* so many times, they have the infographics from these documentaries tattooed on their backs. In fact, vegans often attend special screenings of these films about veganism, clinging onto the hope of one day meeting the great T. Colin Campbell, coauthor of the bestselling book *The China Study,* which examines the relationship between eating animal products (especially dairy) and chronic illnesses, such as coronary heart disease, diabetes, breast cancer, prostate cancer, osteoporosis, and bowel cancer. Dr. Campbell and his son Dr. Tom Campbell prove that eating a whole-food, plant-based (vegan) diet will actually reduce or reverse the development of many of these diseases that are plaguing humankind. They go so far as to write that "eating foods that contain any cholesterol above 0 mg is unhealthy." A vegan diet contains 0 mg of cholesterol. Vegans will also recommend that you watch *Earthlings* (not at all enjoyable) and *Vegucated* (very enjoyable), and, hopefully, they will also buy this book for someone they care about.

Vegans will complain. They don't mean to, but the world is against them. This menu doesn't have enough vegan items. This menu doesn't have the vegan items clearly marked. Why do people continue to look past the cruelty they are committing to animals by eating meat, and why is there milk in nondairy creamer? What exactly does *nondairy* mean then? And, seriously, are you telling me that *all I can eat is rice*? There *must* be more than rice on this menu. Hey, why do these sandals have a tiny strip of leather on them? This list goes on, and ways to adapt to many of these situations are included throughout this book.

Vegans are creative about food. They find replacements for every food they've given up. Eventually, each vegan will eat an authentic grilled "cheese" sandwich or mac and "cheese" or even vegan "bacon." How about french fries smothered in (mushroom) gravy or barbecued pulled "pork"? Even chicken fingers (to this day I'm not sure why they're called that). To make your transition easier and more enjoyable, over twenty-five recipes for many of these replacements are included in the back of this book (page 209).

Vegans will be bold. They make sure they write VEGAN across the front *and back* of any wedding RSVP. They will also call the caterer a few days in advance just to make sure he or she got the message. Then they will mention it when they show up at the reception. To at least two people. And they will still ask when the dinner is served. They often protest the local circus or fur coat store while they wear graphic tees that boldly state: "Vegan for Life!"

Vegans will host potlucks. Many, many potlucks. This provides an opportunity to showcase their new hummus or kale recipes and watch *Forks Over Knives* (again). Potlucks are the vegan's natural habitat and where they feel most comfortable. You will soon assimilate into the underground potluck subculture. Resistance is futile.

Vegans will dehydrate things or annihilate things in their Vitamix. Mostly kale.

Vegans will use soft tofu, ripe avocados, chia seeds, and even black beans. In desserts.

Vegans will not stress about the protein in their diets. Omnivores do enough stressing about this for all vegans—combined. No one cares about another person's protein levels until they find out that person is vegan. Personally, I've never known anyone who has died or even felt slightly weak from a lack of protein. In fact, the only disease directly connected to this is called kwashiorkor, which occurs only in remote areas of famine or poor food supply. If you get enough calories, you get enough protein. How do I know? Vegans told me. Vegans who read the work of people like Dr. Neal Barnard, Dr. Caldwell Esselstyn, and Dr. Michael Greger. Never heard of them? Talk to some vegans.

With the help of this book, you will soon learn *all* the ways of being vegan and merrily mingle among other vegans and help make the world a better place for all beings and the planet. I personally took on a challenge that became a bet to become vegan, and I was as resistant as anyone would be as I was learning the ways of veganism.

I'm now challenging you.

During my first year of being vegan, I was skeptical and very reluctant. But I persevered. Today, I am a proud ethical vegan.

So, lie back in your favorite hammock, crack open a kombucha, kick off your soon-to-be-retired leather sandals, and let's get started on your own journey to veganism.

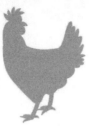

1

THE SKEPTICAL VEGAN: ONE MAN'S TRANSITION TO VEGANISM

It almost seems to me that man was not born to be a carnivore.
—Albert Einstein

It was the best of times, it was the wurst of times. Beef. It's what was for dinner back then. Night after night. The rarer the better. Pittsburgh rare. I used to say to my waiter, "Just lob off the horns and send the cow to my table."

Back then, I was influenced and guided by mass media, the Standard American Diet (SAD), and my own upbringing. Throughout many of those years, I found myself mentored by some pretty amazing university and hotel chefs who taught me proper cooking and grilling techniques, as well as savory recipes that inevitably were plated around meat. The "protein on the plate." If it wasn't beef, it was chicken. If it wasn't chicken, it was pork. Once a year, it was turkey. On Friday, it was fish. I ate shark, octopus, conch, lamb, goat, deer, duck, goose, squirrel, bison, and even bear. If it could be killed, butchered, baked, or barbecued, there is a very good chance I ate it at one point in my life. For the record, and in case this book winds up in the hands of the FBI, I never ate an eagle. At least not a bald one.

The year was 1995. Ithaca, New York. My friend Matthew, a gentle, bearded, tender-bear man with a ponytail halfway down his back, who stood nearly seven feet tall and weighed approximately 280 pounds, heard about a local restaurant offering a Thursday night special: "All You Can Eat Buffalo Chicken Wings. All You Can Drink Beer. $6.95." The Collegetown joint was called The Alamo Restaurant, and ironically, I do remember it.

Back then I was notorious, almost legendary, for my chicken-wing-eating prowess. I was a seasoned "bone cleaner." I could pull the meat off a wing or a drumstick and slurp down the entire hot mess in one bite (while only utilizing three fingers to do so). A friend of mine once asked me to "show him my trick" for eating chicken wings, and I replied, "It's not a trick, it's how you properly eat a wing." I immediately unfriended him.

Matthew and I (also, ironically) walked up Buffalo Street, toward Cornell University, and found our way to The Alamo. We took a window seat overlooking the bustling streets of Collegetown, the miniaturized version of Ithaca's downtown that abuts the Ivy League university. A pimply-faced server approached our table, handed us menus, and introduced himself. "Welcome to The Alamo. My name is Simon. What can we rustle up for you in our chuck wagon, pardners?"

Not looking up, I held the palm of my hand toward the naive teen-age boy and willed the menus away like Obi-Wan Kenobi. "We'll have the all-you-can-eat, all-you-can-drink Thursday night Buffalo chicken wing-and-beer special," I said, with a little drip of saliva finding its way out of my mouth. I was waiting all day to say this, having memorized the promotional poster since Matthew first mentioned it. I ended the order with an Elvis-style "Thank you, thank you very much."

The boy rolled his eyes and walked away.

The waiting was always the hardest part. Anne Morrow Lindbergh once said, "The sea does not reward those who are too anxious, too greedy, or too impatient. One should lie empty, open, choiceless as a beach—waiting for a gift from the sea." She was probably a vegetarian and had no idea about the glory of a chicken wing.

That steamy, crispy, fried outer skin slathered in Frank's hot sauce with melted butter, plunged deeply into a bath of cool bleu cheese dressing. It was about as sensual a food as you could get, and I loved it.

Moments later, the server placed a basket of twelve Buffalo-style wings in front of each of us, along with celery sticks, the aforementioned requisite bleu cheese bath, and a pitcher of beer. Labatt's. The aroma from the steam burned the inside of my nose slightly, and the red orange-slathered skin glistened in the setting Ithaca sun. Matthew and I looked longingly at each other, and then more longingly at the wings. We nodded to each other silently and dove in like Greg Louganis at the 1988 Olympics. By the time the server returned to see how we were doing, we were already prepared to demand our next round. That first batch took roughly five minutes to consume. They didn't know who they were dealing with.

"A dozen more," I said, pointing up my three sticky fingers. The server glanced over to Matthew for his response. He simply nodded and smiled with a trace of wing sauce outlining his lips and signaled for another basket by holding up a single bone. Nothing good was going to come from this.

To the amazement of the server, and management, this went on four more times over the course of a couple of hours until we were finally in the home stretch to consume a total of seventy-two wings. Each. In one sitting. I eventually bowed out at just sixty-eight wings, leaving the last four to escape uneaten. But no less dead than their unfortunate compadres.

The Alamo went out of business the next week.

A year before that, I had made a pilgrimage to the Anchor Bar in Buffalo to visit the site of the original chicken wing. This is where it all started. It was like going to Graceland. This was sacred ground. I often wonder if The King loved chicken wings as much as I did. But I digress.

Now, what I didn't consider at the time, and something that would take almost thirty years to understand, is that seventy-two wings equals a total of thirty-six dead chickens. And when you count how many Matthew ordered and ate, that one fourteen-dollar meal required the hatching, raising, killing, and butchering of seventy-two innocent birds.

Now multiply that by the number of patrons just during that one evening, and you're probably looking at approximately five hundred dead chickens in one small restaurant in small Collegetown up the hill in Ithaca, New York.

Let that sink in.

As a comparison, the national franchise Buffalo Wild Wings sells, on average, twenty million traditional wings each week. Each. Week. That's 260,000,000 (two hundred and sixty million) dead chickens *per year* all from a single franchise. This number is astonishing. And this particular franchise has now opened locations in Canada, Dubai, Qatar, and Saudi Arabia. The carnage is global.

Of course, back in those days, I never once stopped to think about the carnage. I was too enthralled with eating meat. This love for meat eventually found its way into my career.

The midnineties were an exciting time to be an entrepreneur. eBay had just become popular, and websites for online shopping were popping up everywhere. I was sure my friend Mike and I were going to be the next tech millionaires. We had the talent, time, and ability to build an online brand and create a marketplace for a line of products with universal appeal. Move over Internet Shopping Network and Amazon, and make way for MeatBucket.com.

Not even kidding.

MeatBucket.com was your one-stop specialty online shop for everything meat. Your purchase was shipped in a collector aluminum bucket. Customers would visit the site and drop beef jerky, dried beef, smoked boar, Slim Jims, barbecue sauces, etc., into their designer bucket and click "Add to Bucket." They then waited two to three weeks for their meat bucket to arrive. If you acted "now," your order would include a free set of logo toothpicks. Needless to say, MeatBucket.com was even less successful than Pets.com ("because pets can't drive"). We didn't even come up with a sock puppet mascot. But my commitment to meat was clearly evidenced in this project. Meat was part of me. It was as if I were made of meat myself.

Set the dial on the DeLorean ahead another decade to my fortieth birthday celebration. While there were plenty of slender slabs of meat served on skewers, barbecued bits of bite-sized beef drenched in teri-yaki sauce, and bartenders boasting bacon martinis, the highlight of the event was, fittingly, the meat cake. An oversized meatloaf with mashed potato "frosting," professionally piped with gourmet catsup punctuating the perimeter. When that meat cake came out, aglow with candles, I have to admit that I started to cry a little. Not because I had reached a birthday milestone, but because I was so overwhelmed with joy that my cake was made out of meat.

Meat. One hundred percent animal. One hundred percent delicious.

I would eat chicken three nights a week, steak two nights a week, and pork the other two. If there were more days in the week, I'd simply find more meat to eat. If you stop to think about it, there is an endless supply of meat. Right? Keep eating meat, and the meat industry will keep supplying it.

Back in those days, meat meant the world to me, and, eventually, my waistline and heart rate would pay for it.

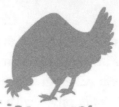

2

FAIR-HAIRED GOLDEN CHILD: THE ONLY SON IN AN ITALIAN HOUSEHOLD

The other night I ate at a real nice family restaurant.
Every table had an argument going.
—George Carlin

Queens, New York. April. Late-1960s. Evening. Peg Anderson Lindstrom had no idea what the following day was going to bring. I was born with a very big head.

I was raised in a half-Italian-half-Swedish household by doting women, sandwiched between two sisters. Essentially, this meant that the sun rose and set on me. The only boy in an all-woman Italian family is treated like royalty and fed as many meatballs and as much pasta, lasagna, ham, and chicken Parmesan as any young man could desire. Italians notoriously eat a lot, but the trouble with eating Italian food is that three days later, you're hungry again.

My mom raised the three of us on her own and worked two jobs—and still always managed to have a complete dinner on the table. Looking back, I'm not even sure how she did this. If I go to the post office and dry cleaners in the same day, I need a nap. She provided for us and, along with her own mom, fed us well. Maybe too well.

Pork chops cooked in butter. Pot roast. Ham. Sausage. Some sort of whitefish. Every meal had meat, and every holiday had extra seasonally appropriate meat. Meat was sometimes found wrapped around meat. Our mom would take us out to Freeport, Long Island, to feed us smoked eel. We would have pickled herring every New Year, a Swedish tradition for good luck, and we would go crabbing in New Jersey and race them on the kitchen floor before dropping the losers, and winners, into boiling water. There were thin-sliced cold cuts in the refrigerator at all times, and, to this day, if you drop by, my mom will have cold cuts waiting. All neatly spread out on the dining room table with sliced cheese and three kinds of bread. And meatballs—we had lots and lots of meatballs.

Oh, and liver. She would make us eat liver. While many people want to believe liver is a "good-for-you" organ, it oftentimes contains poison. Chemical-laden processed feed, antibiotics, vaccine ingredients, pesticide overspray, bad water, and synthetic hormones are mopped up and filtered through the cow's liver, placing it on a long list of animal parts you should never eat. But Mom meant well.

The northern Italian side of my family settled on the south side of Binghamton, New York, a small upstate city approximately three hours from Manhattan, and the current second-place "winner" for the most obese city in America. Currently, the fattest metropolitan area in America is McAllen-Edinburg-Mission in southern Texas, which boasts a frightening obesity rate of 38.8 percent with annual obesity-related costs of over $400 million. And right there in second place was my hometown, Binghamton. With a whopping obesity rate of 37.6 percent and related healthcare costs of over $130 million.

Binghamtonians like to eat, and they especially like to eat meat.

My Nana came to this country through Ellis Island from northern Italy with her two sisters, Mary and Annie. They migrated through New York City, eventually all moving to the south side of Binghamton with the rest of the Italians, most of them getting jobs at the thriving Endicott-Johnson shoe factory. Every Sunday we had the traditional 2:00 p.m. dinner, and every holiday we had unlimited food and stacked trays of cookies. Trays and trays of cookies. Cookies displayed on a tiered cookie rack. My Aunt Annie used to host Christmas Eve at her house, and I'll always remember the place being stacked to the rafters with loud family members, tons of food, all while Aunt Annie's wig watched over us, perched on a foam headstand in her bedroom. She made the worst fried smelt and the best fried potatoes and eggs.

While at our own home or visiting our loud relatives, it felt like we were always eating. It was part of our culture and an opportunity to congregate and spend time together. Italians have traditions of eating small breakfasts, huge lunches, and family-style dinners. We were always eating, and when we weren't eating at home or at someone's house, we were eating out.

At Sharkey's.

Sharkey's is a Binghamton landmark that dates back to 1947 and still stands today. Known for its spiedies, city chicken, clams, and twenty-five-cent bowling machine, its decor is primarily black-lacquer-painted booths, sticky floors, and tacky neon beer signs. I don't think anything has changed at this restaurant since the spiedie sandwich was first invented at Sharkey's just after the Second World War.

Hold it right there. You don't know what a spiedie sandwich is?

The spiedie sandwich. The official food of Binghamton. Marinated lamb, pork, or chicken grilled on a skewer and slid off said skewer with a folded piece of locally baked, thin-sliced Italian bread. Di Rienzo Brothers, represent. For the record, not that I eat the meat version of spiedies anymore, but this is the *only* way to eat a spiedie sandwich.

As a treat, Mom used to take us to Sharkey's for spiedies, all-you-can-eat mussels, and cheeseburger basket dinners as often as her paycheck would allow. The waitstaff consisted solely of a lone ninety-year-old woman who was four foot ten and wore a flower-patterned housecoat. That same old woman is probably still there today, some thirty years later, and she's probably still in her housecoat but maybe only four foot eight by now. We loved going to Sharkey's, and all of us have fond memories of our visits. I'll forever have a little plaque in my heart, technically my arteries, for the place.

Through *all* this, I somehow escaped obesity growing up. But my decadent upbringing of pasta, meat, sweets, cheese, and a barrelful of butter was laying the foundation for the rest of my life. By the time I moved out at age eighteen, I was already a seasoned butter-loving, cheese-eating, infamous animal eater and well on my way to being 250 pounds of solid meat.

I moved out when I weighed only 140 pounds.

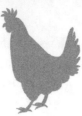

3

MEATY, BEATY, BIG, AND BOUNCY

I always thought filet mignon was the steak to beat,
but the fat content in a rib eye is fantastic.
—*Neil Patrick Harris*

It didn't take long for all that meat to start taking its toll on me. Meat and cheese. And eggs. The Standard American Diet (SAD) represented with a tour of Old McDonald's farm. And on this farm he served a cow, a chicken, a fish, dairy, and eggs.

In America, we eat almost three times as much meat as what would be considered healthy and more than three times as many eggs. But in terms of the recommended amounts versus the SAD ratio? We excel at eating the right balance of one vegetable: potatoes. Root for the potato. Of course, these spuds are most likely delivered in the form of buttered mashed potatoes, salted french fries, and twice-fried potato chips, so they, too, contribute to the poor health of our nation.

And then there's cheese. Americans consume almost eight times as much cheese as even the medical establishment (which is too cheesy to begin with) says they should. Among the major cheese-producing and cheese-consuming countries, the United States was ranked second, with about 10.6 billion pounds manufactured in 2013 alone. Wisconsin, of course, was the leading cheese-producing state with a cheese quantity that amounted to almost three billion pounds that same year. Since 1970, we've gone from eating eight pounds per person per year to a staggering twenty-four pounds!

And add this to your plate: we put more than *ten times* the amount of sugar and refined, processed foods into our bodies.

Americans have become consumed with consuming.

However, for the healthier and more brightly colored vegetables like kale and carrots, not so much. Americans spend nearly 14 percent of their at-home food budgets on sugar and candies, and another 8 percent on premade frozen and sodium-heavy fridge entrées. Whole fruit accounts for less than 5 percent of our grocery bill, and meat is consumed at twice the recommended rate.

And, since I was like every other American, meat was in every one of my meals.

Not only was meat in every meal I ate, but it also made an appearance at most dinner parties, conferences, and events I attended. Starting with a grand tour around the cheese board, it would continue with a few more rounds around the cheese board and eventually become a "build-your-own-pepperoni-and-cheese-stack" competition. I always won. And why did they decorate the cheese board with those pesky baby carrots, cauliflower, and broccoli florets when they were just getting in the way?

Two words back then that I always considered oxymorons whenever I heard them: "portion" and "control." My plate would always be stacked high and to the edges, and I would inevitably go back for seconds or thirds. This attitude was also reflected in the meals I was being served in every American restaurant. A mountain of meat, swimming in sauce, cuddling up against a hill of potatoes, with a garnish of greens.

I never really ate the greens. They're a garnish, after all.

Knowing all this, it's no surprise then that as many as 30 percent of Americans are considered obese. That doesn't include people who are "merely" overweight. While being overweight is bad enough, obesity also seriously increases the risk of chronic illness and death due to diabetes, stroke, coronary artery disease, heart disease, and kidney and gallbladder disorders. The more overweight an individual is, the higher the risk becomes. Obesity has also been tied to an increase in certain types of cancer, but so are meat and dairy consumption even by people who are not obese. We are digging our own graves with our forks and our knives.

While the future of your own health can't be read in the palm of your hand or in the bottom of a teacup, it can in fact be read around your belt.

Now let me be clear that I'm not trying to fat-shame anyone. Nobody should be made to feel inadequate because of their appearance. I'm not saying that Americans who are overweight or obese are blameworthy. What I am saying is that for the millions of people who want to lose weight and be healthy, there is a pretty easy solution: pay attention to the kinds of food you're eating.

Once, I can recall having a physical for a life insurance policy and being told by the nurse that a man's waistline needs to be smaller than his chest measurement. With a simple yellow tape measure, they determine overall health and longevity—and risk.

At that point, both numbers were the same: 40.

If I'm going to be quoted for one thing in this book, let it be this: "Meat, dairy, and eggs will one day prominently display a warning label." This *will* happen in my lifetime, which means it will happen before April 17, 2065 (according to a palm reader at Jackson Square in New Orleans back in 1998). This warning label will not be unlike the one on a pack of cigarettes, and it will look something like this:

GOVERNMENT WARNING: Meat, dairy, and eggs may cause cancer, heart disease, certain diabetes, osteoporosis, and stroke.

Recently, the tobacco-free campaign near me has been plastering buses and running radio ads with the "duh" messaging about selling cigarettes in drugstores. Why would drugstores still sell cigarettes when they also sell the drugs and medications to both help people quit and deal with the nasty side effects and diseases of smoking? Why does my gym give away free pizza and bagels?

Because they have a captive consumer, and making these vices available to them completes the all-important "circle of death." Drug companies (and doctors) rely on sick people to thrive. Health contributes nothing to the global economy.

Let's keep America ill. Abraham Lincoln wrote, "America will never be destroyed from the outside—it will be because we destroyed ourselves."

In 2014, CVS drugstores, an American pharmacy retailer and currently the largest pharmacy chain in the United States, made the very smart decision, in spite of the fact that they turned away billions in revenue, to stop selling cigarettes in all of their locations. The pressure from the public and the obvious disconnect in this messaging led them to this verdict that will hopefully lead other drugstores to follow suit and stop selling cigarettes and tobacco products, as well—a very good move forward toward a healthier nation. Opposition to this is the same as opposition to laws that require people to wear a seatbelt. Some people will complain about their loss of freedom, but most will appreciate the effort and realize it's for everyone's sake. But when will the public, and these very same retailers, make this same connection with meat, dairy, and eggs?

The headline for an article that was heavily circulated the same year CVS made that radical change read: "Diets high in meat, eggs, and dairy could be as harmful to health as smoking." The basic message was written in the headline: *Meat, dairy, and eggs can cause cancer.* When you see someone smoking, you imagine their lungs suffering. When you see someone drinking, you think about their liver deteriorating. But how many people watch someone eating a burger or bacon and think to themselves: "Hmm . . . he might get cancer from that . . . maybe he shouldn't be eating that. . . ." Far too few. It's just not as obvious or apparent to enough people.

We need to stop looking for a cure for cancer and start focusing on its causes. Meat, dairy, and eggs are potentially causing more cancer, diabetes, osteoporosis, obesity, and other horrible diseases than smoking will ever cause; but, alas, you can still buy beef jerky and pork rinds at your local drugstore.

And I used to buy it all.

"Beef jerky, HoHos, and a bag of kettle-cooked potato chips, will that be all?" the ingratiating young cashier asked me as I slid my Diet Pepsi across the counter.

"Diet Pepsi, too."

"Watching your weight?" she asked, as if she were also asking for a throat punch.

"Yeah. Watching my weight," I replied, tossing a large bag of peanut M&Ms onto the counter with my twenty-dollar bill. I was watching my weight as it steadily increased. I kept adding new holes to my belt and new chins to my chin. There was no doubt I had reached "dangerously obese" at that point in my life, and the only way I could deal with it emotionally was by eating more and becoming more overweight. It was a vicious circle, which was also what you could have called my midsection.

I was just like the vast majority of overweight and obese Americans. In the United States alone, the annual revenue of the weight-loss industry, including diet books, diet drugs, and weight-loss surgeries, is $20,000,000,000 (that's twenty billion). This profit-making industry currently serves an estimated 110 million people. Big people are big business. (That last sentence is pretty quotable, too.)

Perhaps, if I knew more about healthy dining growing up, which foods to eat and which foods to avoid, or even this notion of "portion control," I would have . . . oh, who am I kidding? I wouldn't have changed a thing. I was eating like an American, and I was eating to make myself happy—and I really loved being happy.

At one point, when my waistline had finally maxed out at forty-four inches, I hired a nutritionist to consult with me about my diet and weight gain. The clock was ticking, and I knew I needed to lose weight. I was buying new pants and 2XL shirts to accommodate all this newfound "happiness." Eating gave me immense pleasure, and I didn't know how I could stop. I remember buying that first tight pair of pants with a forty-two-inch waist and thinking to myself, "I guess I'm just this big now. This is my size. I'm now fluffy."

My nutritionist had other plans.

"You need to cut down on meat and cheese if you're ever going to lose weight or avoid potentially life-threatening diseases," she said. "And eat more greens."

Before almost falling over with laughter, I replied: "Cut down? Not sure I know how to do that. And does a Shamrock Shake count for 'greens'?"

She went on to explain to me that a single portion of cheese should be no bigger than a nine-volt battery and a serving-size portion of lean meat should be no bigger than a deck of cards. At that point, I was eating a portion of cheese the size of a car battery and a slab of meat bigger than the deck of a cruise ship twice a week. And I wasn't planning on stopping.

Throughout this entire book, I should remind the reader that too much of anything may be too much. That three times the recommended amount of *anything* bad for you is starting from a baseline of already consuming something bad for you. It's not good.

She tried to convince me, through food, that I could enjoy eating healthier by preparing for me balanced meals like a vegan shepherd's pie. Instead of ground beef as the main ingredient, it would be made with lentil beans. Beans. Where do beans even come from? A bean tree?

"Where's the beans?" I quipped as I scraped the mashed potatoes off the top and proceeded to drown them in butter. That meal was basically inedible at that point and tasted nothing like a *real* shepherd's pie. A bunch of beans and vegetables hidden underneath potatoes? No thanks. That wasn't food. That wasn't satisfying. That wasn't what men ate. (As it turns out, my own recipe for vegan shepherd's pie is in the back of this book on page 236. Oh, how people can change. But I'm getting ahead of myself. Back to fat me.)

My pattern of eating not only contributed to weight gain, but also to a few health scares, including heart palpitations in my late thirties. At one point, I went to the doctor with shortness of breath and an accelerated heart rate brought on by climbing one flight of stairs with a basket of laundry. Assuming I was having a heart attack, they ran blood tests, hooked me up to all sorts of high-tech machines, and had me walk on the treadmill for over an hour while monitoring my pulse rate. They poked and prodded me for hours. A team of doctors, clinicians, and skilled nurses hovered over me with their clipboards and stethoscopes, nodding and taking notes and pointing to blinking lights on heart monitors. At my weight, I felt like the *Six Million Pound Man* (which, funny enough, is what they should call *Six Million Dollar Man* in England).

Conclusion after over $800 worth of tests: I was fat and needed to exercise and change my diet.

So, since there was actually nothing wrong with me, I didn't exercise—and I ate more. That'll show those doctors that they're not the boss of my body.

Food—specifically meat, cheese, and eggs—were as much a part of my life as anything. Between hosting elaborate dinner parties or attending Chamber of Commerce events and fancy soirees, I was being fed, literally, my future, one plateful at a time. I was 100 percent sure that if I didn't make some changes, I would be pushing up daisies before I turned fifty-five. At a minimum, I would be on a potpourri of prescription drugs to help "keep me young." I knew I needed to lose weight. And I knew I needed to get my waistline back down to a number lower than my age, but how?

Then, as if sent from heaven, all my prayers were finally answered: *the Atkins Diet.*

A diet so high in protein that all you eat is meat? Yes. Please.

A diet that lets you chew on chicken, partake in pork, and munch on meat twenty-four-seven? Where do I sign up?

A diet that is so effective you can actually watch the pounds fall off your body while giving up none of the palatable meaty proteins my body needed? Out of my way, meat eater coming through.

Dr. Atkins' New Diet Revolution (2002) was the answer to my weight loss conundrum. A revolutionary new diet that recognized, and appreciated, my love for meat. I'd eat three eggs, bacon, sausage, and coffee for breakfast. A protein-packed lunch of cold-cut meat without the bread, and then I'd have a dozen or more chicken wings and a trimmed steak for dinner.

I'd make my body a fat-burning machine.

All protein. All the time.

A "man's diet."

Other male friends I knew had done the Atkins Diet with incredible results. They, too, ate bacon for breakfast, turkey for lunch, and pork for dinner and cut out all those "bad" carbs. One guy I knew only ate steak for two weeks. Three meals that were 100 percent beef. I watched as their pounds were dropping off and knew this was the diet for me.

Over the course of a few weeks, this essentially became the "Chicken Wing Diet." For me, it provided the platform to indulge in my favorite food for all three meals, and the only limiter was how many other animals I could conjure up to consume. The Atkins Diet is also sometimes referred to as "The Lobster Tail Diet," since it included lobster in the plethora of protein-packed proteins you could consume, so naturally I ate more lobster. Dipped in butter. I kept eating more and more animals in an attempt to lose more and more weight. Give me more meat. Drag my knuckles to the all-you-can-meat buffet. Man be caveman skinny. Pound chest, lose pounds. Eat. Meat.

What's not to love about a diet where you eat nothing but meat?

What could *possibly* go wrong?

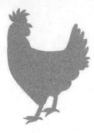

4

FOUR FUNERALS AND A WEDDING

We die only once, and for such a long time.
—Molière

A friend of mine pulled me aside at breakfast one morning. "Pete Watkins is dead."

Back then, my breakfast consisted of two poached eggs on whole wheat toast, sausage, home fries, a glass of chocolate milk, and a coffee. Never deviated from this. Ever.

"Wait? Pete? What happened? He's so healthy," I asked in shock as I shoved sausage into my sausage-eating hole.

"Apparently he was on vacation in Florida with his family and had a massive heart attack while running. He was only forty-eight. It's such a shame."

I looked down at my breakfast, and instead of thinking of Pete or whether or not my diet could impact my health, I wondered if I should have gotten bacon instead of sausage since it seemed "leaner." But then I remembered that I didn't deviate.

"Calling hours are next week. You going?"

Pete was only a handful of years older than I and in excellent shape. A triathlete. How could someone like him die, and die so suddenly?

Maybe it was meat?

Dr. Stanley Hazen of the Cleveland Clinic led a study in 2013 to explore why red meat may contribute to heart disease. Even otherwise seemingly fit and healthy individuals, like Pete, could drop dead from eating too much (possibly any amount of) red meat because of a little-studied chemical called TMAO. For years, researchers had come to the conclusion that what damaged heart function was the thick edge of fat on steaks or the magnetic marbling of their tender lardy sections. These same scientists suspected that saturated fat and cholesterol made only a minor contribution to the increased amount of heart disease seen in red meat eaters. However, the real culprit, they proposed, was this TMAO. As it turns out, a chemical is released by bacteria in the intestines after people eat red meat that is then converted by the liver into TMAO, which eventually gets into the bloodstream and increases the risk of heart disease.

A study looked at six people. It concluded that TMAO was present in five of the meat eaters and not at all present in the one vegan. That one lucky vegan. Pretty sure he told all five of the meat eaters he was vegan before they started the research and then reminded them after seeing the results. The study also found that TMAO levels turned out to *predict* heart attack risk in humans, and they also proved that TMAO actually caused heart disease in laboratory mice (note: not a vegan study). Since Pete ate red meat, and his body reacted in such a way that doctors couldn't easily detect heart disease in time, he essentially had a massive heart attack inside an otherwise healthy body. A seemingly healthy person can die from a heart attack simply by eating red meat.

And it doesn't matter if it's organic, free-range, or grass fed.

By the time Pete's calling hours were scheduled the following week, we all got word that another friend of ours, who was just fifty-four, had also died of a heart attack during a meeting on the golf course. I was in my office when my phone rang.

"Steve died," said Greg, the vice president of our local bank, his voice cracking.

"How? When? My God." What was going on?

"He was on the golf course at the country club. Heart attack. By the time the paramedics arrived, he was gone. There was nothing they could do."

Steve was a pillar of our community and a well-loved man. He relocated to Ithaca from New York City and expected to retire in the Finger Lakes. He and I would dine out together at the country club and talk about future plans. Plans Steve never got to realize.

Later that same year, impossibly, another friend of mine died of a heart attack while water skiing. Robert owned a car dealership. He had a big family and was well respected. I was told that his daughter had to pull his water-soaked, lifeless body out of the water and onto the boat. Unimaginable. He was pronounced dead by the time they reached the shore.

Three men in their midforties and early-fifties, all dying of heart attacks, all within a few months of one another. In 2013 alone, 8.6 million heart attacks occurred in the United States, and it took a total of three of my friends within forty-five days.

Make that four. Amazingly, one more friend died later that same year—of a massive heart attack. Paul was a visionary. An old-school radio guy. A family man. And a friend. He wasn't supposed to die for another thirty or forty years. None of these guys were supposed to die so young.

But they had, and now they are gone.

But not everyone dies young.

When diet is wrong, medicine is of no use.
When diet is correct, medicine is of no need.
—Ayurvedic proverb

As you age, you are forced to pay more attention to all aspects of your health. A couple of years after dealing with the passing of four middle-aged male friends of mine, another friend and a well-loved local radio personality suffered a massive stroke at the station. Geoff was rushed to the hospital an hour away to help stabilize and manage his condition.

Geoff was a heavy-set, big-framed man, but not what I would consider overweight. He ate whatever he wanted and smoked a pack of cigarettes a day. I remember watching him as he put an extralong song on the air so he could step out onto the front porch for a smoke. Combine this terrible addiction with his penchant for fast food, and it really was a matter of time. Geoff was me. I was he. Back then I didn't see what he was doing to himself, and today I am amazed when I see others with these same rituals. Decades of self-abuse that go undetected because they bring joy.

A stroke happens when the blood supply to your brain is interrupted. This choking deprives your brain of oxygen and nutrients, which can cause your brain cells to die. Strokes are usually caused by a blocked artery, which can be directly traced back to meat (and dairy and egg) consumption. It's also been proven that cigarette smoke increases the rate of atherosclerosis. Of course, there are other causes of strokes, but Geoff's diet and smoking combined to create a toxic cocktail that would inevitably lead to a major health complication. The survival rate of people who suffer from strokes depends on how quickly someone reacts.

Luckily, someone was there for Geoff. Geoff's stroke almost took his life, and the entire community was concerned about his well-being. His entire fan base kept in touch remotely on the air and through his wife, who was driving back and forth to the hospital for a week to take care of him. She would send him our love.

In the form of steak. She was bringing him steak. In the hospital. Following a stroke.

Because that's what Geoff wanted and loved, not once thinking it was probably what put him in the hospital in the first place. Humans are creatures of habit, and breaking habits is not easy. I know many friends today who are just like Geoff, and if I told them that adopting a plant-based diet *now* could save their lives, or at a minimum tack an extra five years on the end, they would politely ask me not to force my beliefs on them.

A high school friend of mine also suffered a major stroke at the age of thirty-eight. He is now legally blind and walks with a limp. Steve was never what you would consider a pillar of health—smoking, drinking, and eating whatever he wanted—but he was still way too young to have this happen to him. Steve was one of the reasons I knew I had to eventually get my own life back on track. In many ways, I feared having a stroke more than a heart attack. A stroke seemed less forgiving. More debilitating. Perhaps more painful. I didn't, and don't, want to find out.

Steve and Geoff, like millions of others, were allowing their diets and bad habits to affect their health with each passing moment. They were slowly killing themselves with the very same knife and fork I was using for my own slow suicide.

The only animals I eat are crackers.
—Anonymous

Meat, dairy, and eggs contain cholesterol. This is an inarguable, known fact. If you consume these foods, you are consuming cholesterol, which, in turn, can cause plaque buildup in your heart. While cutting back on these foods, combined with exercise, will certainly add years to your life, in the case of my four friends who have passed and the countless more who are at risk, some may exercise but would never consider cutting back on life's simple pleasures.

If the six hundred thousand people who died from heart disease last year in the United States knew they could be alive today if they had simply cut back on meat, cheese, and eggs or gone on a plant-based diet, would they? Or what about the 150 thousand who die from stroke each year? Are steak and eggs more appealing than a second chance?

Personally, I don't think the majority of people would change a thing—because I wouldn't have, either. By the time an average kid who is fed the Standard American Diet is just *ten years old*, they have already started down the path to forming atherosclerosis in their heart. Clogging of the arteries begins that early and builds up over decades. While many might think adopting a plant-based diet is radical, it's far less radical than open-heart surgery, which is performed half a million times per year in the United States alone. Why is open-heart surgery more acceptable than a plant-based diet? Why don't more people know about the amazing health benefits of a vegan diet?

They're not being told.

Or, worse yet, they are being told otherwise.

Or, even worse, they are being told, and they choose to ignore.

Nearly two-thirds of the United States' economy relies on its population being unwell. Researchers have estimated that by 2030, if obesity trends continue unchecked, obesity-related medical costs alone could rise to $66,000,000,000 (that's billion) a year in the United States. This number is sick. So sick that almost 70 percent of us require costly ongoing medical attention and prescription drugs. From massive organizations dedicated to fighting these diseases to the powerful meat and dairy lobbyists and the pharmaceutical industry that is valued at over $300 billion. These organizations *only* exist if we are sick.

Think about that.

Every employee at any organization dedicated to healthcare, from the CEO to the janitor, relies on Americans being sick. Not well. It's an economic driver of massive proportions. If we are *well*, they are out of business.

A middle-aged friend of mine told me that his primary care physician once asked him what prescription drugs he was on. He answered, "None." To which the doctor replied, "Well, let's see if we can do something about that."

It's a known fact that four out of five doctors prefer an all-expense paid vacation over learning proper nutrition. The fifth doctor in the survey had no comment, since he was busy packing for his annual Pfizer trip to Hawaii. Lured by free pens and golf umbrellas, doctors across the United States reach for the pad and pen long before they focus on the root cause. In fact, some pharmaceutical reps have admitted that doctors have asked *them* what they think they should give their patients. Doctors asking salespeople for advice on what to prescribe.

Doctors are trained to write prescriptions instead of prescribing plant-based diets to their patients. They prescribe medication for many avoidable, and in some cases reversible, serious health issues. In fact, high cholesterol, type 2 diabetes, erectile dysfunction, heart disease, osteoporosis, and others are all manageable by switching to a plant-based diet (combined with regular exercise).

It seems doctors prefer medicating over educating. Think about it. If people heard there was a way to avoid heart disease, most forms of cancer, type 2 diabetes, erectile dysfunction, and possible early death—wouldn't they want to know? Well, consider yourself officially informed.

Your prescription: *Take two pieces of asparagus and call me in the morning.*

And about that wedding? My friend Dave got married that fall, and I was his best man. At that point, I had ballooned to just under 240 pounds. I was officially fat. So fat, in fact, that I was chosen to be a contestant on the (then overweight) Drew Carey–hosted *Power of Ten* TV game show, since we looked so much alike. I remember when I met him on stage wondering if I was *actually* as big as he was. I was. When we were introduced, we just stared at each other, our heads tilted like confused dogs. Maybe we were we just counting each other's chins.

The next six months I spent impersonating Drew Carey around New York, which included my own live stint with Brad Sherwood and Colin Mochrie, two of the stars of TV's *Whose Line Is It Anyway?* I recall seeing their troubled expressions as they sized me up. I thought to myself, "Have I actually become a fat Drew Carey impersonator?"

After one night's performance, a friend approached me and asked where I got the fat suit.

I wasn't wearing one.

That can't be good.

5

TAKING A VACATION
FROM VEGETABLES

*Isn't it amazing how much stuff we get
done the day before vacation?*
—*Zig Ziglar*

For years I would vacation in the Thousand Islands of New York and, by proximity, nearby Canada. If I wasn't sailing, I was fishing. The deep glacier-carved waters are peppered with shoals, and this makes for incredible and diverse marine life. Nearly every freshwater fish is represented in these chilly waters of the St. Lawrence River, and over the course of almost twenty years, I probably caught at least one of every kind.

Muskie. Pike. Perch. Bass. Trout. You name it, I reeled it in.

One summer spent near the shores of Clayton, New York, I caught twenty-nine pike (in addition to nearly two hundred perch, which were bucketed and cleaned to later become "Poor Man's Shrimp"). The pike that I caught ranged from a young six-incher to a whopping thirty-six-incher, which was the most challenging to catch, as it put up an enormous fight until eventually tiring out at the end with a log roll on the water's surface.

This fight, I now understand, is the fish defending itself and trying to stay alive. Taking a fish out of water is their version of *drowning*.

Suffocating. Imagine how terrible it would be to die from being held under water against your will. Pulled underwater by a rope that was shoved through a hole in your lip caused by a sharp knife. You're fighting to stay alive as someone keeps pulling you under deeper and deeper. You. Can't. Breathe. This is how fish feel as they are gasping for the oxygen they filter from water and are brought onshore, or landed in a net. They start suffocating to death.

It's a tremendously stressful, and painful, way to die.

It's oftentimes ignored, or overlooked, that fish have feelings just like any other creature on the planet and deserve to live their lives fully and unbothered. Pescatarians, pseudo-vegetarians who eat meat using "iron deficiency" as an excuse to consume "sustainably sourced" fish, ignore the fact that they are still supporting the industry that nets ninety million tons of wild-caught fish worldwide. These massive fishing operations strip the sea of not only fish during their catch; they also have an irreparable impact on the world's oceans.

I was an avid supporter of the fishing industry for four decades. Everything from sushi to salmon and all the hundreds of fish I caught on my own in between, I *was* a major part of this. From the Caribbean to the Finger Lakes and the Thousand Islands, fishing was my annual summer tradition. While the Thousand Islands boasts some of the best fishing in the world (and, of course, the best salad dressing), they also have their own two-hundred-year-old traditional meal that, ultimately, incorporates much more than *just* fish.

The Thousand Islands Shore Dinner.

This single time-honored meal involves several members of the animal kingdom in its ingredient list: fish, pig fatback, heavy cream, salt potatoes, syrup, eggs, butter, and bourbon.

Fish. Pigs. Cows, Chickens. And booze. All in one meal.

Accompanied by a professional guide, fishermen and tourists who visit the Thousand Islands region have enjoyed shore dinners as a traditional part of the end of a morning of fishing. In the early 1900s, river guides set forth with their fishing parties each morning in a St. Lawrence skiff, rowed by the guide. The guides knew these waters and held the key to the best spots to drop your hook and land a multitude of unsuspecting fish. Fish that do feel pain.

The notion that nonhuman animals might *not* feel pain goes back to the seventeenth-century philosopher René Descartes, who argued that animals do not experience pain and suffering because they "lack consciousness." In 1789, the British philosopher Jeremy Bentham addressed in his book *An Introduction to the Principles of Morals and Legislation* the issue of our *treatment* of animals with the following quote that has been "memed" numerous times by any number of vegans: "The question is not, *can they reason?* Nor, *can they talk?* But, *can they suffer?*"

Tens of thousands of fish populate serene bays that overlook the shipping channels and allow for endless active catches through crystal clear fresh water. The fishing guides would tuck their boats along a rock wall, drop anchor or catch a drift, and help tourists land as many fish as they are allowed to catch.

These salt-of-the-earth guides would then host their own shore dinners on any island that was convenient around lunchtime. After netting as many as two hundred small- and largemouth bass and perch, around noon the guide would call an end to the fishing and head to shore and find a flat campsite to set up the dinner accoutrements for the fishing party to enjoy.

Of course, the fish didn't enjoy any of it.

After the campfire is started, water is put on to boil for coffee, salt potatoes, and corn on the cob that has been stowed on the boat all morning. Along with these and other innocuous ingredients onboard, the guide also stowed a bottle of bourbon and a five-pound slab of pig fatback—a slab of thick fat from a young pig that, when sliced and smoked, becomes the fodder for countless hipster T-shirt slogans.

First to hit the heated skillet is the fatback. Sliced thin, the fatback resembles traditional bacon with one obvious difference. Where bacon or salted pork have *some* lean meat, fatback is just that, 90 percent fat from the back of a pig, with little to no lean meat. This difference is important, at least to the fishing guides and a truly traditional shore dinner. As the fat renders, the residual lard is used to fry the fish *and* the dessert. It is the one "absolute necessity" of the entire production, and for each boat that prepares a shore dinner, there is at least one dead pig who didn't want to be invited.

As the fatback fries, it reduces in size into grease that will be used to cook the meal. When done, the remaining fatty morsels turn golden brown and crispy. A slice of bread, also stowed onboard, is covered with thinly sliced onion, topped with three or four pieces of fatback, and folded into a sandwich. The appetizer is ready for tasting, the first course of the shore dinner. Some have been known to eat more than one of these onion-and-fat sandwiches. I would usually eat five. While I am gulping down the fatback sandwich, the guides would clean and fillet most of the fish, dust them with breading, and put them into the superhot fatback grease to fry. The flesh sears immediately, preventing absorption of the fat (as if that matters at this point, from a health perspective), and in seconds the fish turns golden brown. Meanwhile, in another pot, the fresh coffee grounds that were dumped into boiling water have already settled for more than thirty minutes, transforming the river water into a true aromatic, outdoor delight: black coffee.

Despite all of the things I have given up over the years, black coffee remains. I always feel as though someone who has given up smoking, drinking, meat, dairy, and eggs deserves one vice. And mine is coffee. Good coffee. Black coffee. Gimme coffee.

A vegan friend of mine relayed a funny story to me recently over a cup of coffee. She mentioned that she was on a first date with a man, an omnivore, at a café. She asked the barista to add soy milk to her coffee.

"Soy milk?" he asked.

"Yes," she replied. "I am vegan."

"I'd never go vegan. So, no soy milk for me," the genius added. "I don't want anything made out of beans in my coffee."

Back to that Thousand Islands shore dinner. By now, the salt potatoes have been at a boil for nearly forty-five minutes, and the fresh corn on the cob for ten. It all comes to readiness at the same time, and everyone begins to feast.

While I am eating the freshest fish possible (the very same fish that were fighting for their lives less than an hour earlier), the guide begins preparations for dessert. This is where a shore dinner gets even more interesting.

Eggs are broken into a bowl, and sugar and heavy cream are added. This French toast batter is used for the bread that has been drying in the sunlit river breeze for about an hour. By this point I've already eaten at least five fatback sandwiches and at least as many fried pieces of fish, salt potatoes, and corn, so what could possibly go wrong with something as innocent as French toast for dessert?

Well, the French toast is fried in the same rolling hot fatback grease. But that's not all. Operators are standing by (prepared to dial 9–1–1). The French toast is then topped with butter (of course), a bourbon bottle cap of maple syrup, a bottle cap of cream, and bourbon. All washed down with coffee.

The shore dinner was a 1,300-calorie gastronomic adventure, to say the least.

"Once in your life or once a year certainly won't kill you," a Thousand Islands cardiologist angler was once quoted as saying. He added, "We all eat worse than this and don't pay any attention to it." At least he got that right.

For the record, this same cardiologist is now dead. From a heart attack.

Those days, the cognitive dissonance ran through my blood like spawning salmon toward a waterfall. Summers of shore dinners and suffocating sea life couldn't go on. The meat. The cheese. The butter. Deep down, I knew things had to change.

But change takes time.

> *People eat meat and think they will become*
> *strong as an ox, forgetting that the ox eats grass.*
> *—Pino Caruso*

Every summer when we weren't vacationing in the Thousand Islands, we would sail the Finger Lakes region. We kept our boats at a marina at the north end of Cayuga Lake, the longest of the eleven lakes located in the center of New York State. Hibiscus Harbor is a little-known piece of paradise that was originally carved into the surrounding hills by a quarry. Eventually, it was flooded and became a beautiful and protected marina of almost two hundred boats, ranging from inflatable dinghies to forty-foot yachts. We kept our thirty-foot Hunter there for years.

Weekends were filled with daytime sailing and swimming as well as nighttime grilling and drinking. There was a very rebellious corner of the marina that was well known for hosting the most elaborate parties, and I always took part in the festivities. And the food.

From burgers and dogs to venison and snake, we would take turns bringing new, exotic creatures to grill, or simply wait for a boat to come in with that day's catch. There was always food and drink, and even if the weather wasn't particularly suitable for boating, we all still met to eat and drink and be merry.

One weekend, some boaters planned a clambake. I would provide the rum, and they would provide the clams—wagons full of them. The clams would be grilled until they popped open, succumbing to what could be considered a horrible way to die even for a clam, and we'd then dip the meat in butter and slurp it down. Since they could only grill twenty or so at a time, I began to get impatient and stood over the wagon with a shucking knife and started eating them raw, cracking open each shell and slurping it down with some rum.

This particular event continued until the last person dropped as the campfire turned to blackened embers and nocturnal creatures came out of hiding to scavenge for scraps. These weekend festivities lasted all season long until the crescendo of summer at Hibiscus Harbor sang out over the nearby vineyards.

It was officially time for the annual pig roast.

Hosted by the owners of the marina, this end-of-season event was the one free dinner to thank us all for docking with them. They would provide free beer on tap and two suckling pigs on a spit that would be slow-cooked over coals all day. This was my first experience with a pig roast, and if you've never been, you probably don't want to start now. It's really not the kind of event you show up to offering kale, hummus, and sliced cucumbers, and asking if the potato salad is vegan.

Two whole, intact pigs are wrapped in chicken wire, and a metal spit is pierced through the entire length of their bodies. The hundred-pound piglets are then lifted over the slow coals at 4:30 a.m. to begin their daylong slow cooking. The first year, I woke up at sunrise to watch them prepare the pigs (although I was more likely on my way to bed). The pigs watch you as they are turned by a small electric motor over and over again for hours.

We would walk up to the pigs in the early afternoon and be offered a slice of fatty skin right off the carcass as we crack open our first beers of the day. In addition to the pigs, others bring meat and salads to share, and there is an Elvis impersonator to serenade us as we eat. He ends his set with "Love Me Tender" as he tears off a piece of pork straight from the bone. The event goes into the very wee hours of the morning and, just like every other weekend, only ends when the last person standing has dropped.

It was always me. Lying there, passed out in the grass, surrounded by empty beer cans and half-eaten carcasses.

Meat, in some form or another, had taken control of my life up until my early forties. I never realized just how much, until it also started to take control of my health. I had become a ticking time bomb, and the timer was quickly counting down.

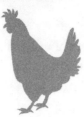

6

WHAT'S THE NUMBER FOR 9–1–1?

Sustained negative flashbacks can stir a heart attack.
—T. F. Hodge

I lay there on the living room couch, my left shoulder and arm in such intense pain that I couldn't sit up. My head dug into a pillow as I was finally ready to succumb. I couldn't bear the pain anymore and knew I needed to get to the hospital.

Earlier that day was the first day of my new workout routine. Time to get into shape. Patrick, a scrappy Irishman, had trained prize-winning boxers, and he himself was the epitome of great shape. Every year he would run as many miles as his age, with as much weight on his back. I met him when he was forty-eight and running forty-eight miles carrying forty-eight pounds.

Patrick was what I needed.

I needed discipline.

I needed a routine.

I needed to get in shape.

I needed an ambulance.

Instead, I got a ride from a friend to the local convenient care and checked myself in, all the while bracing my left arm, trying my best not to move it.

When a man who is my age and weight checks in with severe pain in his left arm, they take it pretty seriously. In the United States, someone has a heart attack every thirty-four seconds, and every sixty seconds, someone in the United States dies from a heart disease-related event. I was probably the next to go.

Think about that staggering statistic and then read this next paragraph slowly and out loud:

> Meat, dairy, and eggs contribute to heart disease. There are delicious and healthy plant-based alternatives to each of these foods that contain zero cholesterol and *won't* contribute to obesity or the hardening of my arteries that potentially could lead to a fatal myocardial infarction (heart attack) as well as a massive stroke. As I was reading this paragraph, someone in the United States just had a heart attack.

I was checked in at convenient care within minutes and immediately rushed into one of the private suites and hooked up to every conceivable contraption to monitor my vital signs and stabilize my condition.

"How's the pain?" A nurse asked, checking my pulse and lowering the back of the examination table to a full reclining position and unbuttoning my shirt. She pointed to a cartoon poster of the pain measurement scale.

The first face was smiling and the caption read, "Zero. No Hurt." The last face was red and sweating and cringing from pain, and the caption read, "Ten. Hurts Worst." Under that caption read, "Worst pain imaginable."

"That last guy," I said. "Worst. Terrible. Excruciating. Please give me something."

I pleaded, just wanting the pain to subside enough to see straight. It was as if someone were digging an electric soldering iron into my shoulder and wouldn't stop.

"Doctor will be right in," she said reassuringly, yet doing nothing about my red, sweating, and cringing condition. She stepped out into the hallway to find a doctor, and I overheard her say to another on-call nurse, "I think he's having a heart attack."

I yelled from the room, "I'm not having a heart attack!"

Or was I? How should I know? I've never had a heart attack. No one in my family has ever had a heart attack. We live forever.

Well, not exactly forever, but damn close. My Nana died at ninety-three in her favorite armchair at home, tea steeping, reading her Harlequin Romance novel, and waiting for Jeopardy to come on. She passed away peacefully after a full afternoon at work feeding other senior citizens, some thirty years younger than she, pizza fritte. Her two sisters lived well into their eighties, and my mom is a fit seventy-five-year-old. We are sturdy stock.

A few other clinicians had passed my room when a young doctor entered and asked me a series of questions as he continued to examine me and flip the pages on my chart. All the while the pain was continuing to intensify. It had become unbearable.

"Can you give me something? Please? Make the pain go away," I begged.

The doctor left the room and came back with two pills in a small cup and another cup of water. He instructed me to take the pills to help ease the pain but said I shouldn't plan to go anywhere anytime soon. I took them since I had no plans at that point anyway. I was in too much pain to sit through a movie or go out to dinner; I was probably right where I needed to be.

I shot down the medication. Within fifteen minutes the pain subsided. All the while more nurses were coming in and out, wondering what to do *with* me and if there was anything else they could do *for* me.

After an hour had passed, the drugs started wearing off, and the pain began to slowly return. Since the resources were limited at the convenient care and the doctors were still concerned I could be having some version of a heart attack, they insisted I get admitted to the nearby hospital. By this time, my original ride who had driven me to convenient care was already asleep, so I was left with no choice but to be transported via ambulance. A thousand-dollar, fifteen-minute ride for a heart attack I wasn't having. Or was I?

At the hospital, the medic whisked me into an ER room. Because of my weight, he required the assistance of three other people to lift me onto the examination table. I had become someone who would have to plan for at least six pall bearers. I was too heavy to tandem skydive, that's if I would be allowed to fly on a small aircraft in the first place, and I was too heavy to bungee jump, since I'd probably take the bridge with me.

More nurses hooked me up to even more elaborate equipment and kept checking my blood pressure and asking me to choose a face on the pain chart. A few minutes later, another nurse came in and began tapping my arm to find a vein to insert the IV.

"What's going on?" I asked, his thick needle inches from my right arm.

"We'll take care of you, just relax," he said, plunging the needle into my arm, swinging around gracefully, and hanging the IV bag on the infusion pole. He turned back to look me over.

"On this scale from one to six, with ten being 'unimaginable,' what number would you associate with the pain in your arm?"

"Get a new poster. I'm off the chart," I said, because it was true. Or, maybe I was being a baby. Since arriving at the hospital, the pain had intensified. It started in my shoulder but with the passing hours had moved farther down my arm. Is this how I'm going to die? In a hospital? What happened to my plan of jumping my motorcycle over Snake Canyon through a circle of fire?

"Any chest pain?" he asked, now tightening the blood pressure cuff over my arm. "Do you think you're having a heart attack?" he asked, all the while pumping it up.

"A what? No. I just pulled something while working out this morning. That's all."

Trying to get back into shape got me into the emergency room. It was the black fly in my Chardonnay.

Another older doctor came in and examined me. Peering over the top of his glasses, he asked me the same questions the two doctors before him had asked and insisted I was having a heart attack. This went on for three more hours until a shift change brought in another doctor who would finally become the last doctor I would need that night, and my savior.

"Where's the pain?" he asked, squeezing my shoulder to make me wince. This doctor was different. He was a tall man. Handsome. Mustached. If this book is made into a movie, I recommend Tom Selleck play him. (He'll have to grow back his mustache, though. Seriously, why did he ever shave that off? Or Alex Trebek? What were they thinking?)

I winced. "There," I said, pointing at the joint in my left shoulder through tears.

He reached into his cowboy holster and pulled out a needle that was six inches long and held it up against my skin. Maybe Clint Eastwood could play him, if he were younger.

"This is going to hurt like hell. Brace yourself," he said as he plunged the needle into my shoulder joint and began moving it around, injecting every corner with cortisone.

"The pain should go away in . . . three . . . two . . . "

"One," I said with an exhale and a relieved smile. The pain was completely gone. Dr. Magnum, P. I., was a genius. He gave me a pat on the back, lifted me upright into a sitting position, and handed me a glass of water.

"We'll have you checked out in a few," he said, holstering his needle.

Turns out it was only a pinched nerve. Not a heart attack. I pulled something while working out on the very first day with my new trainer. I had been trying to tell them all along, but they weren't listening, or maybe they just couldn't hear me through all my crying and whining.

But what I didn't tell them was that it happened while lifting an eight-pound weight. Something had to give. I knew I couldn't go on like this. My life was half over, or half not over; I couldn't tell. Either way, it was too much. Too much of *everything*.

And not enough of Jen.

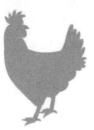

7

MEETING JEN
AND GOING VEGAN

Where there is love there is life.
—Mahatma Gandhi

It took eight attempts to get Jen to finally accept a date with me. Eight feeble and hilarious tries via messaging on a popular online dating site. After eight of my best pickup lines and pseudoromantic come-ons, she finally agreed to go out with me. She admitted that I was not her type and didn't really want to meet me. Spoiler alert: she's stuck with me now. For. Ever.

Our first date was over dinner. Jen has celiac disease, an autoimmune disease where she can't consume gluten. She was also vegetarian at the time. So, for this meat-eating, chicken wing–worshipping, pizza-loving aficionado, choosing one of my usual hangouts was probably not going to go down too well, literally. I left it up to her to make the recommendation.

"Have you ever eaten Korean?" she asked in a text message as I was getting ready, dousing myself in five-dollar cologne and Brylcreem-styling less hair than I think I have.

"No," I texted back, although at the time I would have assumed that Korean food was similar to Japanese food, which was just like Chinese food—and I've eaten tons of Chinese food. I think this way because I am a white man in America. Besides the numerous nights of delivery and takeout Chinese food, my mom used to make chicken chow mein all the time for me and my two sisters.

"Sounds great. See you at eight."

When I was eighteen, I moved out of the house and went away to college. I had to cook everything in an electric frying pan since I couldn't afford to turn the gas on in the third-floor apartment I was renting. Hungry one night, I climbed into my 1982 red Chevy Chevette (I used to tell girls I drove a red Vette) and navigated my way to the local grocery, which wasn't that difficult since Nanticoke, Pennsylvania, has one traffic light and one grocery store. I browsed the shelves for a while until I spotted it. It. There on the shelf, next to the instant boxed rice, was a can of La Choy Chicken Chow Mein with vegetables, sauce, and dried, fried crunchy chow mein noodles. Already homesick, I was excited to buy it, and, of course, it met the minimum requirement for meals I could make at college: it could be cooked in an electric frying pan.

I quickly drove home from the store, blasting a cassette tape of Elvis Costello, smoking a cigarette with my window down in February. The window handle had broken off a week earlier, and I didn't have the money to fix it. I felt like Kevin Bacon in a British-pop, emo, small-town Pennsylvania sort of *Footloose* way. The big town rocker with the can of chicken chow mein and the electric frying pan.

Dashing up the stairs to my apartment, I quickly plugged in the pan and turned it up to the highest setting. I deftly opened the cans, poured the contents into the heated pan, and stirred it up with the one wooden spoon I owned. Looking back, I now wonder if that was the same wooden spoon my mom would smack me with. She had probably sent it to college with me to subliminally keep me in line.

My first real meal away from home, and I was destined to make something just like Mom used to make. I spooned the hot chow mein onto one of the two plates I owned, added the crunchy noodles on top that came in the taped-on, attached can, and took my first bite.

It tasted *just* like Mom's.

It tasted just like *home*.

I ate the entire serving and, with a belly full of food and a heart full of love, ran downstairs to the bar on the first floor to call my mom. Back in those days, I would have to call collect from a payphone. I dialed zero plus one plus the twenty or so required digits to put the call through, and she picked up.

"Hello?" Peg said. My mom always knew just what to say at just the right time.

"Mom, it's Eric. Your son." I was her only son, and she knew it was me since the call was collect, but I still liked to announce myself. "You're not going to believe this! I made my own dinner tonight. Went to the store, bought a can of La Choy Chicken Chow Mein, and cooked it in the electric frying pan. It tasted exactly like your recipe! I am so happy!"

Long silence.

"You dummy. That's what I've been feeding you kids all along."

Like I said, Peg always knew just what to say.

Meanwhile, fast-forward some twenty-plus years into the future to a dimly lit Korean restaurant in Ithaca, New York.

Jen had suggested Four Seasons, an authentic local Korean restaurant near Cornell. She could indoctrinate me to Korean cuisine and order her favorite dolsot bibimbop, all while keeping an eye on the door in case she had to make a run for it. We sat in the window seat, and I stared blankly at the menu, which was mostly in Korean. It was at this moment I suddenly realized that *perhaps* all Asian cuisine is not the same. Jen sensed I might be struggling.

"What do you like?" she asked, leaning in, probably trying to steal an extra whiff of my cologne. I could tell I was growing on her. I looked fancy, had great hair, and I was saying all the right things. As the consummate conversationalist, I answered her question with a one-word question.

"Meat?"

"Okay," she said. "How about this?" She pointed to an item on the menu, and of course I had no idea what it was.

"Sounds good!" I replied.

The waitress approached and Jen placed our order using an intoxicating mix of English and Korean. Within a few minutes, I was served a steaming skillet of meat. Korean bulgogi. Essentially, it's a huge, hot serving of thinly sliced marinated beef piled high and cooked to just under medium, with rice and gochujang, Korean hot pepper paste, on the side. She also ordered me a bottle of soju, Korean rice liquor that's so incredibly smooth you hardly notice what you're drinking—and back then I probably drank a few.

I dug into the meat with metal chopsticks and didn't slow down until it was gone. It was delicious. So meaty.

Our conversation swirled from "What do you do?" to "What movies do you like?" and back around to talking about food.

I looked at my skillet where the pile of meat used to be, the half-empty bottle of soju, and then looked up at Jen. I was falling in love.

We married two and a half years later, six months after becoming vegan together. We eloped to downtown Chicago.

Jen grew up in a suburb of Chicago. We had decided to take a long road trip to this amazing Midwest city to spend time there and see the house she had grown up in. On an impulse while in a traffic jam, I asked Jen to look up what it would take to get married in Illinois, and, as it turned out, we had everything we needed in the car with us. And, since her parents and brother were planning to come to Chicago that weekend as well, why not get married?

At that point in our relationship, we were living together and were certified foster parents with the hopes of adopting a newborn. I knew I would never find anyone as amazing and inspiring as her, and getting married was the most romantic, spontaneous, and best decision I've ever made in my life.

Still stuck in traffic while driving into Chicago, we wrote our single wedding vow (spoiler alert): *To be vegan for life.*

> *Becoming a vegan was the biggest change I ever made in my life,*
> *and one of the greatest accomplishments as well.*
> *—Woody Harrelson*

Every so often you meet someone who has a profound effect on your life. Often, these people have no idea that you've chosen them as mentors;

they go on with their amazing lives doing amazing things without ever once stopping to think about you. Rather rude of them, I'd say.

Some people look up to God. *She's* awesome. Others choose the Dalai Lama. Sharp dresser. Still others might be inspired by the Queen of England. I've got money on her living to be a million years old. Or perhaps Abraham Lincoln, inventor of the luxurious and reliable Lincoln Continental.

That last one might not be entirely accurate. I may have to Google that.

Meanwhile, some people choose a jackass. Those people are me.

Just before Jen and I went vegan, I met the man who would unknowingly help to forever alter the course of my future: Steve-O. Professional Jackass.

As it turns out, Jen went to high school in London with Steve (they actually attended senior prom together), and they've remained friends ever since. When Steve toured the country back in 2011 with his stand-up routine, Jen and her high school friends decided to hold a mini-reunion in Washington, DC, to watch his show. Jen met up with Steve and some other friends for brunch the morning of his performance to catch up on old times. I decided I would crash their brunch and meet the man himself.

I was never really a Steve-O fan, per se. I think I'd watched a few episodes of *Jackass* and probably watched the first *Jackass* movie, but that was about all. Through Jen, I learned he was sober *and vegan*, and I found that fascinating. Of all people who would be one of these things, let alone both, I wouldn't have pegged Steve.

Steve has had so much of his illustrious past and wild personal life caught on camera—and today he's proud to be clean, sober, and vegan. Unrelated, but no less fascinating. I also happen to know that Steve abstained from sex for more than four hundred days, which, to be honest, seems much more challenging to me than going vegan.

Steve, Jen, and their high school friends were seated at a very busy Busboys and Poets in downtown DC and were fairly easy to spot. Say what you will about Steve; he is a celebrity and was continuously surrounded and interrupted for autographs and photos by adoring fans. I should mention that Steve's famous for being very generous in providing photo opportunities to anyone who asks and ends every one of his stand-up shows with a *very* long line leading up to a personal Steve-O selfie moment.

I sat next to him and watched him eat as everyone else caught up on the years they spent in London and traveling around Europe, summing up the two decades that had passed. A young hyperventilating woman timidly approached our table and asked Steve if she could get a photo with him. He lit up with a smile and agreed; her day was made. This continued throughout the brunch until he finally had to start asking people if he could please finish his tofu scramble before taking any more photos. Which he did.

According to Steve, back when he was doing cocaine and nitrous, he started hearing voices in his head that told him he would have to "answer" for his cruel actions. Then, he heard a Krishna Consciousness guy ask in a YouTube video: "How can you expect to be saved if you eat meat?" Steve became terrified of having to answer for all of the suffering he was causing animals and, after a short stint at being a pescatarian (a vegetarian who eats fish), he finally went vegan.

Less than a month later, Johnny Knoxville and the other Jackass crew staged an intervention for Steve for drug and alcohol addiction. While in recovery at an undisclosed rehab facility, Steve was introduced to the idea of replacing fear with faith (or love) and made an effort to follow this path. He soon realized he was happier as a result of practicing more compassion. Further proof that people go vegan for any number of, and for their own, reasons. Even voices in their heads.

In more recent years since that brunch, Steve has become more of an outspoken vegan and a powerful voice in the community. He narrated a video for the not-for-profit Mercy for Animals that has been viewed more than a million times, and he has a unique and loyal audience that is *listening*. He is using his celebrity to make a difference for the animals and to promote veganism, somewhat passively, through his millions of followers.

As I creepily stared at Steve that day, chewing on his hash browns and laughing about his high school antics, I had an epiphany.

If Steve could go through everything that he had up to that point, make the same incredible life changes he had made, *and* be an ethical vegan on top of that, then I could. *Anyone* could. And should. I was starting to feel like I needed to make similar changes in my life, at a point where it could still make a difference.

We left brunch and toured the nation's capital, stopping to take a photo of Steve posing with the Washington Monument as a placeholder for his penis until he finally had to duck into a cab to avoid being molested by fans.

It was that day I decided I would become a jackass.

Not really. I already am one, but Steve helped bring that aspect of my life into focus and inspired me to think about my own future and try to make positive life changes. While the idea of being vegan wouldn't officially present itself for one more month, meeting Steve factored into so many other positive changes that were about to happen.

> *Being a vegan just helps me build up my self-esteem.*
> *I feel good about it every time I eat a meal.*
> *—Steve-O*

A few years later, we met with Steve for lunch at the vegan Strong Hearts Café in Syracuse, New York. We talked about that weekend in DC, his stand-up show, his world travels since we last saw him, and he told us some fascinating stories about being vegan. Stories about the challenges of being vegan on the road. Stories about vegan setbacks and stories about establishing and maintaining meaningful relationships when your partner isn't vegan. Stories about how others view veganism and animal rights.

Stories that suddenly made sense to me.

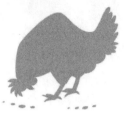

8

THE BET: WOKE UP VEGAN

Horse sense is the thing a horse has which
keeps it from betting on people.
—W. C. Fields

December 2011. Jen ordered a copy of Colleen Patrick-Goudreau's *30-Day Vegan Challenge* after hearing our friend Sherry talk about the book at the vegan, gluten-free, macrobiotic Friday dinner we attend. Sherry's precocious ten-year-old daughter, Meena, cornered us and told us that we "should be vegan." This best-selling guidebook for getting started in veganism sat on our kitchen table, in plain sight, for a few days before Jen told me her plan.

"I'm going to do this," she said, handing me the book. "I'm going to go vegan starting on the first of the year."

I remember looking at the softcover book and was reminded of a friend of mine. Jaime was a four-foot, ten-inch fireball who used to drink with the boys. We would go out to the usual haunts, load up on chicken wings and beer, and let loose. I remember when she told me she was vegan. At that point in my life, I had no idea what it meant to be vegan, and she was the only vegan I had ever met.

"I don't eat meat, dairy, or eggs," she yelled over the loud house music while we were dancing at The Haunt.

"Are you serious?" I yelled back. For the sake of the rest of this conversation, just assume we are yelling back and forth to each other while dancing. "What the heck *do* you eat?"

"Fruits, vegetables, lots of salads."

"And no meat?" I asked, troubled by this.

"Tofu."

"No meat?"

"No meat."

"I can't even. I'd starve to death."

"It's not bad. Great for your health. Vegetables are good for you!"

"You're like a Salad Shooter," I joked. Laughing hysterically at myself for coming up with that. The idea of not eating meat or cheese was so foreign to me and so against everything I stood for, I couldn't believe I actually knew someone who did not eat meat or cheese. What a weirdo. Who would do something like that? You'd have to be crazy to give that up.

I looked back at the *30-Day Vegan Challenge*. The cover claimed it was "The ultimate guide to eating cleaner, getting leaner, and living compassionately."

Why would anyone go vegan?

I couldn't answer this simple question. I had no idea of any of the health benefits or the positive impact a plant-based diet has on the environment, and I had little to no sympathy or compassion toward animals, with the exception of cats and dogs and a goldfish I named Chomchi.

I took the book, opened it, read some of the chapter heads. Flipped through some of the recipes, and then stopped and thought about the past forty years of my omnivorous life, my own health scares, my weight issues, my age. Thought about Steve. And Pete. And Geoff.

Then I looked at Jen. She had already been vegetarian for years, so taking this step was not a big stretch. She already felt she was lactose-intolerant, so eliminating dairy from her diet would make her feel better overall. She wasn't fond of eggs, only eating an occasional egg on her bibimbap. She was already accustomed to a restricted diet because of celiac disease.

I was an omnivore with very strong leanings toward carnivore.

I was an animal eater. I loved meat.

But I loved Jen more.

"I'll do it with you," I said a couple days later, not at all knowing why in the hell I said it or what I was thinking at the time. Could I somehow take it back? Maybe she hadn't heard me. In the back of my mind, I thought: *It's only thirty days. I'm sure after thirty days we'll both go back to our usual diets and lifestyle, and we'll regift the book and move on.*

"What?" she asked, with a somewhat doubtful but supportive tone.

"Sure. It's only thirty days. It'll be fun."

Those thirty days weren't fun.

We had travelled to Arizona to spend the holidays with her parents, and we told them of our plan to go vegan. Of course, we were telling them the plan over a steak dinner I had prepared. I believe the steak was drowned in some sort of béarnaise sauce, and the dish probably included a side of meat.

One of Jen's college friends had also gone vegan the year before. When we visited her for two weeks in Arizona, she cooked for us, shared recipes, and bragged about how going vegan had made her feel the best she'd ever felt physically in her entire life. Her husband claimed to be 98 percent vegan (whatever that meant). Apparently, he still ate baked goods that contained butter and eggs. Spending time with them in Arizona gave me some confidence that I could stay vegan if I wanted to—though I didn't know if I wanted to.

Arizona allowed me to "consider" new food choices and "get a feel" for being vegan, while still enjoying my usual meals. Jen would order soon dubu, a Korean soft tofu soup, and I'd order it with beef. She would get a gluten-free pizza loaded with veggies, and I'd get mine loaded with meat. While I was considering the new food choices I was about to make, I wasn't going to go down without a fight.

Meat was the Thelma to my Louise. The Jack to my Diane.

But all of this was about to change dramatically.

I'll never forget the night before the first day I went vegan. We were traveling through the Newark Airport. A banner the size of a bus was promoting a chicken wing special at some greasy airport restaurant.

One thing to note about me and my illustrious history with chicken wings: I would find the good in any preparation of a chicken wing meal, even if it was from a gas station.

Especially if it was from a gas station.

The banner was calling my name. We had a layover. We had to eat. The special was a limited time offer. The banner was so beautifully designed with so many wings, perfectly cropped and airbrushed like a Victoria's Secret model. As we got closer to the restaurant, the scent was erotic. Calling my name. I was drooling.

Jen noticed the drool.

"Are you gonna go for it?" she asked.

All sound in the world stopped for one second.

"Nah," I replied. My body felt like it was possessed by Sally Struthers, or someone else who never has any fun. "I may as well start now," I continued. "Why put it off? I'm vegan."

To this day, I occasionally awaken from a sound sleep with a racing heart, sweat dripping off my forehead, chewing on my pillow, thinking about that banner and those uneaten wings.

We made it home safely and went straight to bed. Fell asleep a meat eater and woke up vegan.

Day one quickly passed, and I successfully avoided meat (or cheese or eggs). *I got this*, I told myself. If I manage not to eat all meat, cheese, and eggs for just thirty days, on day thirty-one I'll host a BBQ with other carnivores and run around barefooted, beating our chests and wearing fur. Even though it would be February in Upstate New York.

Within the first week of being vegan I had a business lunch with a potential new company I was considering working for. The owner and CEO invited me to meet at a popular Ithaca restaurant, and I thought, "Here I go, set out into the world as vegan."

Would people stare at me? Would they know I was vegan? Would I get a knowing nod from other vegans as I walked down The Commons? Do I have to start wearing Birkenstocks with my business casual attire?

Pat and I sat in the window seat, and I explained to him that I was a one-week-old vegan, that this would be my first attempt at ordering food, and that I hoped he would be patient. The server came over and asked what we wanted.

Pat immediately ordered straight off the menu. I, on the other hand, was lost.

One by one, we went over every item to see which had nonvegan ingredients. Little things like egg in a sandwich bread or dairy in a salad dressing were popping up in item after item. It turned out, after ten minutes of trying, that the only thing I could eat was a salad that was custom-made for me by their accommodating chef.

Total cliché. The vegan orders a salad.

When Pat asked me why I was vegan, I shrugged it off and let him know it was a passing thing and I really wasn't planning to commit to it 100 percent. Early vegan denial syndrome.

Within a few minutes, Pat's beefy sandwich, slathered with beef and dipped in beef juice, appeared and filled my nostrils with the aroma of beef; and my salad, covered in salad, was placed in front of me. I quickly inspected it, my eyes darting to Pat's lunch, and dug in. This was only thirty days, right? Not a day longer. I can last thirty days eating rabbit food. Radishes, and greens, and carrots, and tomatoes . . . and walnuts.

Damn, walnuts. They had put walnuts on my salad, and I'm highly allergic. Figures.

The server came back to make sure everything was all right just as my throat started to close. Pat said yes while I nodded without opening my mouth.

The rest of the meeting, I drank water to alleviate the reaction and played the strong, silent type for the interview. It must have worked, since I ended up getting the job as the new vice president of marketing and communications for a million-dollar construction company—who is vegan.

Hours turned to days and days turned to weeks. Before I knew it, three full weeks had passed. Twenty-one days. Somehow I was still alive, in spite of the fact that I should have been dead weeks ago from an apparent protein deficiency. Looking ahead another week, I realized I could actually make it. The thirty days were nearly over. Piece of vegan cake.

It was time to make this challenge interesting.

"What are we going to do after thirty days?" I asked Jen, while most likely gnawing on a carrot or celery stick. I was now an expert at grazing.

"Keep on keepin' on."

"Then let's make this a real challenge. A bet," I blurted. I think being vegan for thirty days made me blurt more often than I used to.

Not even sure why I blurted. To extend the challenge even further was insane, but I thought I could win this thing. I knew that Jen missed cheese, and I have amazing willpower. Plus, I love a good challenge.

"Okay, you're on," she said. "What are we going to bet?"

My first instinct when my wife asks, "what are we going to bet," is always sexual favors, but that was vetoed, so we agreed that the loser would have to do all the chores for three full months. *All* the cleaning, laundry, housework—everything—while the other sat back and relaxed. And, of course, the winner could gloat while eating a chicken wing pizza. That was going to be me.

I knew I would win The Bet.

So, *all this*. All my veganism—a lifetime of no meat, dairy, eggs, or honey—started with The Bet.

The Bet that, to this day, I refuse to lose.

A full thirty-one days into being vegan, and something felt different. I ate an entire breakfast and felt . . . great. Full without feeling sick. As if I had just eaten a vegan cloud of happiness surrounded by edible flowers. My traveling companions on another business trip were all experiencing stomach pains and frequent trips to the bathroom following their hearty bacon and cheese omelet breakfasts while I ate oatmeal, fruit, and black coffee—and felt content. Was I onto something? Could being vegan really make you feel better? About yourself and about your choices? Forget therapy, give me broccoli.

I was already getting into a pretty good rhythm with my diet. Eating whole grains and mostly plant-based foods with the occasional veggie burger or fake chicken patty thrown in. We were also experimenting with other "replacement" foods to satisfy my cravings: pizza with Daiya vegan cheese, tofu wings, sweet potato fries, soy curls, and other delectable vegan treats that aren't great for you but taste great.

It was at this point that something magical came into my life.

A vegan friend of mine texted me asking if I had ever heard of Beyond Meat. He was coming back from a protest, or some other vegan event, in the Washington, DC, area and had brought back some of this new "fake" chicken meat. Up until then, there were some nice options, but nothing had the same texture and taste as real chicken. He was raving about it, so I was eager to give it a try.

He met me behind the local food co-op, like some sort of vegan drug deal, handing me a mason jar of leftover Beyond Meat.

"You're going to freak out when you try this," he said.

I ran home and pulled out the strip of "meat," sniffed it (for the record, I smell everything before I eat it), and gave it a try.

To this day, I don't know if I will ever experience the level of euphoria I experienced in that one bite. That one moment in my vegan journey was the beginning of a turning point. Maybe the light at the end of the tunnel wasn't a train after all. It was isolated pea protein molded into the shape of a grilled chicken strip, and it tasted and felt just like chicken.

In my opinion, Beyond Meat changed over-the-counter vegan meat substitutes forever. To this day I remain Super Fan #1 (true; actually, you can find me on their website). They recently rolled out the Beyond Burger, which is the closest thing ever to a "meat" burger I have ever tried. It bleeds beet juice.

It was also at this point in my life that I was finally finding my groove in the kitchen and adapting many of my old recipes into their vegan counterparts. Yet dining out remained a challenge. As I was finally starting to feel some of the positive effects of eating vegan, it was time to venture out to see what else I could eat in the "real world."

"Do you have anything vegan on the menu?" I asked the blonde server at my formerly-favorite chicken wing slinging bar and restaurant. I wasn't optimistic and figured I would settle for a salad, minus the meat, cheese, and dressing once again. Her response, on the other hand, felt like angels flying down from heaven and sitting next to me in my booth for a lunchtime snuggle. And by "angels," I am referring to the original *Charlie's Angels*, especially Kate Jackson.

"For the most part, no. However," she leaned in. "I'm vegan, and I've come up with my own off-menu meal. I think you'll like it . . . assuming you like french fries."

I may have found heaven on earth. Veganism *was* possibly going to work for me.

The meal was everything I'd dreamt it would be. Big juicy veggie burger and crispy french fries. All vegan. Proof that I could still frequent some of my favorite places, only needing to work with the server or management to make it happen. I started thinking that all those other vegans were right. This *could be* an excellent way to live.

And then I had my annual physical.

Nothing will benefit human health and increase chances for survival of life on Earth as much as the evolution to a vegetarian diet.
—Albert Einstein

I had already given blood to the lab so we could immediately discuss the results at my annual physical appointment. That morning at the doctor's office, I stood on the scale and weighed in at 212 pounds (I had lost more than five pounds in the first sixty days without even trying) and proceeded to sit across from my doctor to discuss my numbers.

I am at an age where most doctors are expecting dismal numbers. They usually line up their prescription pad in preparation for what ails you. In place of a stethoscope they have a ballpoint pen. They've examined enough overweight fortysomething men to know that it's all downhill from here.

Or uphill.

"Hmm. Your cholesterol," she said, reviewing the numbers and cross-checking with greater scrutiny, "has *dramatically* improved: HDL is 53 and LDL is 70. Pretty much cut in half from your last visit." She looked at me as if I'd done something wrong or I had somehow Ferris Buellered the data. Checking my blood pressure, she said, "Perfect. 110 over 60. You seem to be doing something right." My pulse rate was 70, my weight was going down, and I passed the rest of my initial exam with flying colors.

"Whatever it is you're doing . . . keep doing it," she remarked.

Oh, I'll keep doing it, I thought as she gloved-up for the prostate exam.

"I have to," I replied, lying on my side as she poked around my prostate for proper size or any abnormalities, easily my favorite part of my annual exam. I have a very nice prostate, I've been told. "There's a lot at stake. Or was it *steak*?" I winked. Probably shouldn't have winked at my doctor during a rectal exam.

The benefits of being vegan were starting to show in more ways than one, most noticeably when I fastened my belt a few weeks later and had lost four inches in my waist. Plus, there was The Bet.

Getting rid of my old leather belt and replacing it with a vegan one had now become a necessity for keeping up my pants. Friends of mine of the same age were all fattening up and swallowing down whatever pills they needed in order to continue with their current lifestyle, while I had discovered the Fountain of Youth.

I was actually shocked at one point during the first two weeks of being vegan when a close friend of mine told me his doctor had prescribed him a pill that he could take every day to keep his arteries clear enough so he could enjoy as much meat and dairy as he liked. He was delighted to know that keeping on this one drug meant he could eat as much butter-drenched, bacon-wrapped steak as he wanted. Not at all considering the possibility that he might have a much shorter time than he was originally planning to do so, and not acknowledging that this drug was brought to his attention only after his own father had suffered a stroke.

And, of course, with no mention of changing his diet. It's easier to stay well prescribed than *well*.

I began really paying attention to what I was eating and what impact it would have on my own health and the planet. I had always been one to think that one person couldn't make a difference; but, suddenly, I was feeling like I may have found my groove. My purpose.

Now, don't get me wrong here. As much as I was enjoying the benefits of a meat-, dairy-, and egg-free life, I was still dreaming of chicken wings. I was still the outcast at the company pizza party. I was still longingly looking at the glistening images of burgers that floated across my TV screen. I was still an omnivore at heart and was still hoping (against all hope) that Jen would eat *one* slice of cheese. One *morsel*.

And lose The Bet.

I am constantly reminded of a cartoon I once saw: two Tyrannosaurus rexes are standing over the grill as a Brontosaurus walks up to the cookout. The brontosaurus announces, "I brought hummus!" to which the T. rexes reply: "Who invited the herbivore?"

Was this all worth it? Was being a restaurant's worst nightmare the way I wanted to live? Would I ever stop dreaming about chicken wings?

Then I watched the documentary *Forks Over Knives*. Not since *Porky's* has a movie had such a long-lasting, profound effect on me. Seeing the evidence and hearing the results a plant-based diet so prominently presented helped make this short-term bet into a potential life-long decision. Additionally, actually meeting Dr. T. Colin Campbell, a leading authority on plant-based nutrition, in person and hearing his assurances that, over time, I would feel even more health advantages helped convince me that I could be onto something.

That night, I had another chicken wing dream, only this time the chickens were still using their wings, flapping around their roost, and I was happily eating massaged kale. Oddly, dressed in a chicken suit.

Still not sure what that was about.

> *Eating meat is the most disgusting thing I can think of.*
> *It's like biting into your grandmother.*
> *—Morrisey*

When you first go vegan, you may notice that your hair starts to thin or fall out, your skin begins to break out in bumps, and your teeth suddenly become more sensitive to cold. You may also suddenly feel fatigued. Rest assured, not one of these symptoms is a result of going vegan. Some of them may be a result of imbalanced nutrition, but none of them can be blamed on veganism.

It's like saying your face muscles are aching from smiling.

Veganism isn't a diet. It's a lifestyle. Within this lifestyle, you're avoiding meat, dairy, and eggs, and any dramatic diet change is going to have some effect on your body.

Over time you will find the right formula and the right balance. You will most likely have to supplement Vitamin B12 and possibly Vitamin D. Vitamin D can also be easily absorbed by spending time in the great outdoors, perhaps petting pigs at a farm sanctuary or rescuing turtles on the side of the road.

The health benefits of being vegan often take time to kick in as your body adjusts to no longer eating what you've eaten for the better part of your life—patience is key.

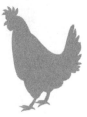

9

ON BEING SKEPTICAL: GOING ALL IN

People don't resist change. They resist being changed.
—*Peter M. Senge*

And there I was. Vegan.

For the first half of my life, I could eat anything I wanted—so I did. Didn't matter what it was, where it came from; if it had eyes, fur, fins, or parents. Didn't even matter if it was served still moving. I would eat it. The world was my oyster, so I ate them. Raw. Washed down with lemon and horseradish. Now I wasn't even sure I could *eat* horseradish, since I didn't know if it came from horses.

My diet took a 180-degree turn. From Meatville to Tofutown. I had a one-way ticket from Porkland, Maine, to Portland, Oregano. I have no idea what that means, but at that point in my life, I excused myself for irrational thinking.

But what had I become? Why did I agree to this challenge in the first place, and then make matters worse by turning it into a bet? A bet that could have lasted a month, maybe two, and no more than three. Jen really loved cheese.

Well, apparently, she hated housework more than she loved cheese. By now, almost a full year had passed. Three hundred and fifty days.

There I was. Still vegan.

I soon found myself surrounded by other vegans and talking about vegan things. Would I have to one day help them protest the circus? Would I host another screening of *Blackfish* if they brought the popcorn covered in nutritional yeast? Did I get a chance to read that amazing new book about all the incredible benefits of a whole-food, plant-based diet by Dr. McBoringguy? Was I getting enough B12? What was B12 anyway?

Obviously, I was in this all the way, and it looked like I wasn't coming out of it any time soon. In between moments of clarity, I still experienced moments of doubt. It was a rough first year with many ups and downs.

Two months into being vegan, I was really missing a lot of the food I used to eat. Burgers, wings, fried shrimp dipped in ranch dressing. Then there was Pizza Day at work. God, I missed pizza. It was like a gooey, cheesy, pepperoni-covered, foldable cigarette. Only the cool kids ate pizza. I was eating carrot sticks. I didn't belong.

Friends were sending me recipes to tease me. Deep-fried gravy. Bacon-wrapped French toast strips. Beer can chicken. Igloo meatloaf. The national advertisers on every TV network were out to get me, tempting me with cheese-drenched burgers, sizzling sliced steaks, and meat-topped meatballs. All filmed in slow motion and backed up by porn music. Bow chicka wow wow.

Online ads. Radio ads. Billboards.

Everywhere I turned. Meat.

> *Could you look an animal in the eyes and say to it,*
> *'My appetite is more important than your suffering'?*
> *—Moby*

"My Name is Eric and I'm a Omnivoraholic," I lamented in front of a room full of total strangers.

"Hi, Eric." The reply in unison was ominous, but what did I expect from a group of vegans who now consider themselves "recovering omnivores?" We were all once meat eaters. Milk drinkers. Egg scramblers. We knew what one another had gone through, and what the future held. This was never going to be easy.

"It has been just over a year since I last ate meat." Reflecting back, the last time I ate an animal, it was probably chicken, in the shape of wings. Or maybe it was a meat lover's pizza. Or was it a sirloin steak? Just thinking about it made me hark back to those "good old days."

I knew I had a problem when I saw wing sauce drippings on my bed sheets. Once, I had a half-eaten bologna sandwich in my back pocket that dripped mayonnaise into my leather wing-tips. I had hit rock bottom.

And that's when I found Omnivores Anonymous (OA) and learned about the twelve-step program for quitting meat, dairy, and eggs for life. We learned we were powerless over those three ingredients. But mostly cheese; so many of us fell off the wagon because of cheese.

We came to believe that a power greater than ourselves could restore us to sanity. His name was Joaquin Phoenix, and his lifetime commitment to veganism was legendary. We made a decision to turn our wills and our lives over to fruits and vegetables and embrace a vegan diet. We cleared our closets of wool, silk, and leather, even though I loved our Limited Edition Tommy Bahamas Pool Ball silk shirt, and, at the same time, we cleared our arteries of gunk and goo and our guts of fat and poo.

We experienced a spiritual awakening. We carried this message to other omnivores and committed to practice these principles in all our affairs. We knew it was in us to grab hold of our own destinies, to clear a path to better overall health.

But, most important, we knew it had to be done . . . for the animals and, in my case, for The Bet.

A friend checked in on me on day fifty of being vegan.

"How has it been going? Do you feel better or any different with this food challenge?"

"Food challenge? You mean torture, right?"

I was in and out of touch with reality, and still skeptical at this point. "Day fifty . . . I feel . . . almost *exactly* the same! That's kind of the let-down right now. I am going to go a full six months and see if that has as positive an impact as I was 'promised.' If not . . . look *out* all you chickens, cows, pigs, flightless birds, fish, gerbils, cheese wheels, ice creams, and reptiles! Bet be damned!"

"Make sure you eat plenty of birch bark salad with a side of twigs," she joked.

I wasn't laughing. I was counting. The minutes. The days. The weeks. After a full two months of being vegan, I reported back to her: "Being vegan is wonderful! Except for the whole 'not eating meat, fish, cheese, and eggs' part of it."

Maybe this wasn't going to work for me after all.

And maybe Jen wasn't going to eat cheese.

Yet still I refused to lose The Bet.

"One to change a few. A few to change many.
Many to change the world. Starts with one."
—Anonymous

Early on into my veganism, Jen custom-ordered me a black T-shirt with the words "Reluctant Vegan" in white letters centered on the chest. I loved it. It was me. My preferred way to dress has always been all black anyway. My fashion sense is second to nun. This simple black shirt was perfect—I was forever mourning the loss of meat in my life. This shirt was either eventually going to be retired forever because *she* ate cheese and I won The Bet, or it was going to be worn by me forever as a reminder of who I had become. I wore that simple black shirt everywhere, notably to Friday Dinner.

Friday Dinner. The hidden hippy place to eat on the outskirts of Ithaca, if you wanted to partake in a gluten-free, vegan, macrobiotic dinner. (No, I didn't know what macrobiotic meant either. Big food? Big organic food? Food covered in macrobes?) The place where people consume pressure-cooked brown rice with chopsticks for some odd reason and sprinkle their food with some sort of sawdust. Where people chew every bite one hundred times with their eyes closed.

I wore my black "Reluctant Vegan" shirt to "Patchouli Central."

"You're not reluctant anymore," one of the crunchier vegans said, noticing my new magic black shirt as soon as I walked in. Taking off her shoes for dinner and handing me a cup of hot twig tea with two hands, she went on. "You know you love it. Being vegan."

I heard nothing. The magic black shirt cancelled out all that noise.

The magic black shirt had superpowers. It could shield me from all the vegans while re-attaching me to the omnivores. *My people.* It made a bold statement about who I was.

"I'm not planning on being vegan forever. I love meat too much." Was that out loud? I might have said that out loud.

I took my favorite seat at the far end of the table and puffed my chest out, creating a billboard, waiting for the reactions from all the vegans in the room. Wanting them to come at me with all their veganism. Call me out. Defend themselves and defend the animals. Try to tell me I was one of them. I was ready for it. I was prepared. I had the magic black shirt.

"Nice shirt," Mike said, with a chuckle.

And?

Nothing. Crickets. Tumbleweeds.

I looked around the room. Fifty or so vegans happily interacting with one another. Laughing. Eating. Splashing wheat-free tamari in their soup. Going on with their own vegan lives.

No one else noticed or cared. How could that be? I was blatantly broadcasting my indifference to veganism, letting them know this was not something I was planning to continue. Didn't they see this? Didn't they know what the word "reluctant" meant?

I sat there, quietly eating my gluten-free, macrobiotic, vegan dinner washed down with twig tea—sulking. In my magic black shirt. Which maybe wasn't that magic after all.

World Peace begins in the kitchen.
— Anonymous

Over time, people accumulate stuff. Things. Belongings. Some save very little and some are hoarders. Trust me when I say that when you go "all in" with being vegan, you're better off having very little to start off with.

Turns out, there is a bit of leather in pretty much everything.

When I decided to go vegan, I decided to go "all in." You don't have to; you can still wear your leather sneakers or wool sweaters or silk boxers, but the likelihood of being called out by an omnivore is incredibly high. Imagine being cornered in an alley by a gang of animal eaters, pushed up against a brick wall, and barraged with questions like, "Hey, vegan, where do you get your protein?" "Would you take antivenom if it meant saving your life?" And then they glance down to see your leather wingtip shoes. Or belt. Or watchband.

I wanted it *all* gone. I wanted to prove to myself, or not, that I could be 100 percent vegan. (Plus, I didn't really look good in my assless chaps.) I went through my closets and drawers, packed a massive box, and gave my clothes away to friends and the Salvation Army, or sold it online. Not at all unlike giving up meat, dairy, and eggs, I was suddenly giving away clothes that I loved, including lounge shirts made from silk, and silk comes from silkworms. And silkworms *are* animals.

Mass-produced silk comes from domesticated silkworms that are raised on silkworm farms. Today, China and India remain the top two producers of silk. The silkworms, while in the caterpillar stage of the silk moth, are fed mulberry leaves until they're ready to spin cocoons and enter their pupal stage. The silk is secreted as a liquid from two glands in the caterpillar's head. So far, this doesn't sound terrible, and it's what nature intended silkworms to do—but it goes south from here. While the silkworms are still in their pupal stage, the cocoons are dropped into boiling water, which kills them and begins the process of unraveling the cocoons to produce the silk thread.

They are boiled alive to extract the silk threads. Your silk sheets, underwear, neckties, shirts, and scarves are all made from silk that is derived in this way. If the silkworms weren't boiled alive, they would turn into moths and eventually chew their way out of the cocoons to escape and fly—free. Or free to fly into a hot porch light and die. But that's not the point. They chose that path themselves.

I rid myself of all my silk, leather belts, boots, wallets, and shoes. It all had to go.

Even my beloved motorcycle jacket. For a while, I owned an Indian Motorcycle and had to have a flashy motorcycle jacket to match. An extra black, with extra straps and snaps, biker jacket. It matched my *meaty* persona. I have no idea how many cows were sacrificed for that jacket, but it had a lot of leather on it.

After I sold the jacket online, I later sold my bike. Neither seemed to go with my new *vegan* persona (though, as far as I know, the bike wasn't made of meat or cheese or eggs).

As you take inventory of your own life and belongings, keep in mind that transitioning to being vegan takes as much or as little time and commitment as you'd like. Changing your diet to vegan is pretty straightforward; selling your Land Rover because it has a leather interior is going to take some thought. Take your time.

Each day you spend as a vegan, you will grow more and more attached to its core beliefs and less attached to your stuff. A friend of mine held onto her belongings for sentimental reasons and, one day on her own, decided to give away the nonvegan items to other family members to cherish.

I also watched a vegan YouTuber who, for years, presented herself with her abundance of belongings, all of which were, in fact, vegan. One day, she decided to get rid of it all. She realized she just had too much stuff and simply let it *all* go. Downsized. Feng shuied. Simplified her wardrobe and her belongings. Immediately, she felt more connected to herself.

In my case, I had no sentimental attachment to anything (with the exception of that Tommy Bahama shirt, which now belongs to a coworker). It was easy to switch over to vegan versions. I found amazing vegan shoes that I still wear nearly every day, as well as a vegan belt, vegan jackets, and even vegan lounge shirts. Meanwhile, I am writing this book on a computer that is clearly not vegan (because the screen contains animal-derived material). The tires on our hybrid car are not vegan. Plastic bags contain "slip agents" that are derived from animals. White sugar is often filtered through animal bones, and I'm sure there are many other things hidden in my life that are not vegan.

But I am doing the very best I can and would never go against being vegan intentionally. Being vegan simply means I am trying to suck *less*.

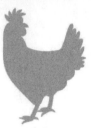

10

FRIDAY DINNER

The hippies wanted peace and love.
We wanted Ferraris, blondes, and switchblades.
—Alice Cooper

Early on in my relationship with Jen, before we were both vegan, she told me about a vegan, gluten-free, macrobiotic dinner in Brooktondale, about ten miles from downtown Ithaca. Ithaca itself is a rather "hippy" small city with bumper stickers that boast being "ten square miles surrounded by reality," and this is pretty accurate. Ithaca has its own currency, which is good for one hour of work and can be traded among local residents who are likely adorned with dreadlocks and sandals. This Ithaca money will buy you a cup of coffee with one hour of reiki massage. That's so groovy.

Ithaca also holds the record for the largest human peace sign.

In 2000, Ithaca's residents pulled more ballots for Ralph Nader than for George W. Bush, and this number would have been even greater if Nader had paired up with Dennis Kucinich. In 2016, Ithaca was the single largest financial supporter of Bernie Sanders, all from a city with fewer than fifty thousand full-time residents. Home to the influential hippie eatery Moosewood Restaurant, Ithaca is also the headquarters for the Namgyal Monastery—a branch of the personal monastery of the Dalai Lama—as well as the location of the Dalai Lama's library and

Kurt Cobain's ashes. Residents are required to have a minimum of ten bumper stickers supporting social and environmental causes plastered across their Priuses, Subarus, or beat-up Volvos.

Now, drive fifteen minutes outside of town; it can only become even more earthy-crunchy and more off-the-grid (drive another forty-five minutes, and you're in a completely *opposite* world).

This is where Friday Dinner is held.

Back then, I still had no idea what *vegan* meant, let alone *macrobiotic*. A macrobiotic diet consists of whole, pure, prepared foods that is based on Taoist principles of the balance of yin and yang. The food on your plate has its own energy. And you thought *vegan* was hippy?

According to macrobiotics, the broccoli on your plate has its own energy that can be absorbed by the sweet potatoes, which will channel its vegetable karma into your millet patty. Or something along these lines. A properly planned and plated macrobiotic meal is perfectly balanced, so as you eat it, complete with mismatched chopsticks, you can use the food's yin and yang to heal all that ails you. Of course, for it to really work, you also need to chew each bite a hundred times.

However, if watching a bunch of hippies eating their food very slowly with chopsticks while humming "mmmmmm" is what ails you, you may want to avoid Friday Dinner.

Friday Dinner takes place in a humble home in Brooktondale, New York, and it has been happening for more than twenty years. Every Friday night, Priscilla and Lewis open their hearts and their door to their home and serve a homemade gluten-free, vegan, macrobiotic three-course meal to any number of regulars and whoever else finds out about it from secret underground channels. Or their website.

It was at this first Friday Dinner that I was about to get indoctrinated fully to the vegan lifestyle. Me, with all my metrosexuality, eating dinner shoeless in the country with a bunch of hemp-wearing weirdos. Weirdos like T. Colin Campbell, the noted nutritionist, co-author of *The China Study*, and featured talking head in the films *Forks Over Knives* and *PlantPure Nation*. Yeah, he goes to Friday Dinner.

You can't miss the house, since there is a four-foot-high peace sign that is lit up, cutting through the country darkness, nailed to the side of the house. Country darkness is the darkest darkness, and this sign is a beacon calling out to all the hippies. In the country, no one can hear you scream.

Jen wanted to share this with me, so I agreed to tag along, not knowing what to expect, but hoping they had free Wi-Fi and a full bar. Turns out they have a wicker basket by the door to drop your twenty-dollar suggested donation into, and that's about as high-tech as it gets.

We walked up the wooden staircase into an enclosed porch adorned with a pile of shoes as a colony of hippies congregated over the twig tea and water station. Twig tea. Since twig tea is composed of the stems and young twigs from the tea plant, it is rich in both vitamins and minerals that feed the leafy parts of the plant. Hippies love it. They hold their hand-tossed mugs with two hands and breathe it in. They make "mmmmm" noises when they take a sip. I have no idea what they do with the actual tea *leaves*, maybe smoke them, but twig tea tastes like just tea. All the vegans mill around, sipping twig tea and talking about solar panels, living off-the-grid, or the book they are reading or writing.

I stood out in this setting as I was still trying to connect my iPhone to a Wi-Fi signal—or any signal, for that matter. Send help.

After finding a seat at one of the many folding tables and making nice with introductions, Lewis, a slender, high-energy man, led the room in a moment of quiet reflection. We all held hands. Everyone closed their eyes. But not me. I didn't trust these people.

We were asked to breathe in. *Breeeeeeathe innnnnnnn.*

My eyes darted around. What's next? A chorus of Kumbaya? Not exactly, but close.

Lewis then instructed us on the proper technique of blessing the evening's meal, which culminated in a clumsy attempt of everyone trying to say "blessings on the meal" in unison.

After the blessing, Lewis launched into a very animated live rendition of the night's menu. Loudly and enthusiastically announcing each of the courses and many of the ingredients (forgetting one or two along the way and encouraging the "audience" to help him remember actually added to his routine). I am not sure if any other restaurant in the world does this, but I was pleasantly surprised by the opening ceremony.

"Let's see . . . we're having millet cakes . . . and pressed salad . . . and brown rice . . . and butternut squash soup . . . and . . .," he went on, finally ending with dessert as the whole room mmmmmed again in harmony. Everyone then settled in, waiting for the first course to arrive.

And the small talk began.

"Are you vegan?" a woman with wiry gray hair and thin glasses asked me as she sipped her twig tea, holding it with two hands, before proceeding to choose a suitable set of chopsticks with which to insert her yin and yang into her vegan pie hole.

"No, I'm not," I replied nervously.

"Why not?" she continued. She seemed like the kind of woman who would continue.

"I like chicken wings too much," I said, probably too loudly for this room, but there was no way I could take it back. It was out there. The six words *I like chicken wings too much*, mixing with the aroma of patchouli and simmering quinoa, was pretty much how I introduced myself to the rest of the table at Friday Dinner.

"So," she started, her eyes directly locking into mine. "You *enjoy* animal cruelty?"

Wait. What? What did she just ask me? If I *enjoyed* animal cruelty? Who said anything about animal cruelty? I just mentioned that I love chicken wings. Didn't she know who she was dealing with? I once ate sixty-eight chicken wings in one sitting. (Unsurprisingly, every time I see this woman nowadays in my postvegan era, she corners me about finding her a vegan man. Hit me up if you know anyone.)

The rest of the dinner went as could be expected. Awkward small talk about veganism, upcoming vegan potlucks, vegan events, vegans in the news, etc. I was uncomfortable, out of my comfort zone, and not impressed.

Until I ate the food. I have to admit, the *meal* was incredible. It was unlike any meal I had ever eaten before in my life.

Every meal at Friday Dinner starts with soup. In all the years I've attended, I've never once had a bowl of soup I didn't love. Soup is such a warm and welcoming way to start a meal. Each bowl is plant-based, some containing just three simple ingredients, and yet they explode with a depth of flavor and texture you'd never expect.

Following soup is the entrée, a plate *loaded* with a variety of offerings: pressure-cooked brown rice, kale salad, pressed salad, nori rolls, tempeh, tofu, and other seasonal (mostly local) fare. The plate is alive with color and flavor, and it's always very satisfying. In fact, all the food is so good you completely forget it's gluten-free, vegan, and macrobiotic.

While many of the diners who attend are, in fact, vegan, some are vegetarians, some are raw foodists, and some are omnivores, like I was when I had my first experience. These unsuspecting meat eaters are somehow coaxed into attending and eventually find themselves enjoying a meal they might not ordinarily try. A three-course, cruelty-free meal for twenty dollars.

To this day, it remains the only meal I've ever had that includes a shaker of gomasio—a mashed up blend of sesame seeds and sea salt—on every table. It looks like sawdust, but it's really good on just about everything. Or, as the hippies say, "mmmmm."

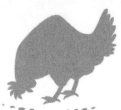

11

THE TRAVELING VEGAN; OR, A VEGAN IN A MINNESOTA STEAKHOUSE

The world is full of magic things,
patiently waiting for our senses to grow sharper.
—W. B. Yeats

I'll never forget driving through the Pennsylvania countryside one crisp fall afternoon and gazing at the grazing cows peppered on the bucolic hillside. For my entire life up until this point, cows (1) provided milk and then (2) became meat. Or, if I wasn't in the mood for milk, they were just meat. These monochromatic mammals roam about the countryside by the thousands, waiting to be milked or killed. Milked or killed. Milked or killed.

There really isn't an in-between for cows.

Very few farmers keep cows as pets, but there are many farm sanctuaries that do. A farm sanctuary is a place where animals who have been abused, neglected, or abandoned in commercial farming institutions can live out their lives in a peaceful environment, where they are cherished and properly cared for. Animals in "factory" farms often collapse under the pressure of their failing health and agonizing living conditions. They don't receive the medical attention they deserve because it is cheaper to let them slowly die. So-called grass-fed, humanely raised, free-range cows don't fare much better. The tiny fraction who are fortunate enough to enter a sanctuary can leave this nightmare behind and live out their lives fully.

There are more than 1.6 million cows living in Pennsylvania alone who are destined for a life of slavery and abuse. Nearly two million animals grazing the frackin' hills of the Keystone State.

In fact, I was once so inspired by the ever-present herds of helpless heifers that I launched a marketing concept that sold advertising on the *sides of cows*. "Cowvertising" would allow companies to have their logos spray-painted onto the skins of these animals. The thinking was: They are already standing there anyway. Cowvertising brought an unheard (unherd?)-of new meaning to the phrase *corporate branding*. With over a million and a half roaming billboards in Pennsylvania alone, I was expecting to go public within the first year.

Needless to say, Cowvertising eventually went out to pasture.

Now, driving with my window down and my hand cupping the cool country air, I could inhale the aroma of the meat and dairy industries hard at work. With each inhalation, I felt alive. *Appreciating my own life.* The difference was, on this particular day I was also contemplating *their* lives. Something I had *never* done before.

These cows are sentient beings, I thought, with emotions and feelings not unlike humans. They love and nurture, show joy, and socialize. According to research, cows are generally very intelligent animals who can remember things for a long time. Animal behaviorists have found that cows interact in socially complex ways, developing friendships over time, and sometimes holding grudges against other cows who treat them badly. They are not there for us to use.

Most important, they have a will to live.

What was *happening* to me?

What was this feeling that was coming over me?

I pulled over to the side of the road as three cows slowly moseyed their way to the barbed wire fence. As they got closer with each step, they became more *real* to me. More approachable. I wasn't seeing steaks, I was suddenly seeing personalities. Animals who were curious. Animals who wanted attention. Animals who loved fresh country air as much as I did. Animals who had offspring they loved, cared for, and nursed.

That is, until their offspring are suddenly and violently taken from them.

A pregnant cow carries her young for nine months. After nine months, she begins to experience contractions and labor pains. She endures tremendous discomfort during the birthing process and watches her newborn emerge—and, as with any animal, she has unconditional love for her calf, her offspring. Cows often exhibit emotional distress when their calves are taken from them and bellow for hours or even days. In Sarah Taylor's book *Vegetarian to Vegan*, she cites a story about British neurologist Oliver Sacks, who visited a dairy farm with Temple Grandin, a professor of animal science, only to hear the "very loud and unnerving sound" of cows bellowing. Grandin suggested that the farmers must have just separated the calves from the cows, and it was indeed the case.

Sound familiar?

I stood there motionless as cars whizzed by me. Almost apologetic. Overcome with some sort of guilt for what I had done in my past. It was at this moment that I was truly "making the connection" I had heard about from other vegans. It was then that I knew there was truly no turning back.

All bets were off.

I got back in my car and probably passed another few dozen dairy farms until I made it to my office. All I could think about were those animals and their well-being. While so many openly grazed the rolling hillsides and seemed content in the morning sunlight, I was horrified to think about what was happening behind closed doors, inside the barns and at nearby slaughterhouses.

Newborn calves stolen from their wailing mothers within a few hours of being born so humans can take the mother's milk. Older milking cows, no longer able to be impregnated or no longer lactating after birth, slaughtered for meat. A literal endless cycle to satisfy an omnivore's palate.

I walked up the flight of stairs into my office and proceeded to boot up my computer. Opening Facebook, I noticed a friend had invited me to an event that weekend in Buffalo. The "9th Annual Beer and Bacon Festival" poster appeared on my timeline, featuring a lineup of musical acts, food vendors, beer sponsors, and a headline that I couldn't shake. Couldn't ignore. I simply couldn't process the thoughtlessness of the message: "Now with More Pig!"

What have we become as a species?

When did we become so callous and heartless? When the benefits of veganism are *so* evident and animals are *so* innocent, how could we continue doing what we were doing? And why haven't so many others made this connection?

> *When you feel the suffering of every living thing*
> *in your own heart, that is consciousness.*
> *—Bhagavad Gita*

One Friday night during my first official year of veganism, I ventured out to Friday dinner by myself.

Jen stayed home with Baby #1, and I headed out to the country to enjoy a healthy plant-based meal on my own. As it turned out, a mutual friend of ours, who is a vegan nutritionist, was also present, and she brought three friends. All omnivores.

I sat at the head of one of the long tables in my usual seat, flanked by these four young women, two on each side. I thought to myself, *This is a nice head of the table—intelligent, beautiful women to talk to while eating a healthy dinner among plant-loving allies.*

But I had no idea how wrong I would be. How *ugly* beautiful could become.

Soup was served. Broccoli tofu noodle soup. Everyone praised the first course, the bowls were collected, and soon the conversation turned to a plant-based diet and veganism.

"You do know that humans evolved to eat meat, right?" one of the Cornell University-educated seniors whispered to me. Whispered loud enough to let me, and everyone around me, know she wanted attention.

"What?" I asked, almost embarrassed for her, or perhaps the feeling was more one of wanting to kick her under the table. In a room full of peace-loving vegans, she wanted to start something? She wanted to go "there"? Hadn't she ever heard of militant vegans?

"We are meant to eat animals. Always have been and always will be. Our teeth are made for eating meat. All animals that have teeth like ours eat meat. So, we should be able to eat meat." She took a sip of the soup and looked me straight in the eye.

Never before had I met someone with such conviction. So much confidence in her message. So much chutzpah! It was as if she were planning this attack during the almost thirty-minute drive from the city just to corner an unsuspecting vegan. And she had chosen me.

"Are you speaking from a health perspective? Because that could be argued against," I replied, looking at the far end of the table for any sign of support from my fellow vegans. Nothing. They either couldn't hear this conversation or assumed I could handle myself. I thought of signaling to them by holding up an SOS napkin but decided I wasn't about to involve them in what could possibly become a productive conversation. I was ready for this. I may have been the Skeptical Vegan at one point, but I also knew enough to hold my own.

So, I didn't send for reinforcements. And the conversation didn't become productive.

"Our brains formed because of meat protein. A diet with no meat goes against how human beings evolved," she continued. Our friend, who is vegan, smiled at me as if to say, *Have fun with this one.*

"She's right, you know," yet another one of the matching blondes chimed in. They were a gang. But I was prepared. The Sharks versus the Jets. The T-Birds versus the Scorpions.

Time to throw some plant-based shade. (By the way, arugula, beets, broccoli, brussels sprouts, cabbage, carrots, cauliflower, celery, chard, Chinese cabbage, corn salad, endive, escarole, garlic, horseradish, kale, kohlrabi, and leaf lettuce are all shade-grown vegetables.)

"Actually, a whole-foods, plant-based diet is optimal for excellent human health. Obesity, certain diabetes, some cancers, and especially heart disease can all be controlled, and sometimes reversed, on a plant-based diet. Dr. T. Colin Campbell, Professor Emeritus at Cornell, has published volumes on this subject and is living proof that a diet without meat, dairy, and eggs, is the healthiest." Boom. Take that.

Short silence. Her eyes began to twinkle. I may have had her up against the ropes. Until she said, "*Don't* get me started on animal rights."

Where did *that* come from?

"Humans are more intelligent and more rational than nonhumans. These characteristics give us the right or opportunity to be able to use nonhumans for food. Therefore, we should be able to eat meat. Animals are a commodity. Livestock is raised to feed humans." I started to lose my appetite. She continued, "My father happens to be the number one provider of pork to a well-known national grocery chain. If you walk into any of their fifty locations, his photo is displayed in the deli. He is pretty much the man who is responsible for all the pigs in a five-hun-dred-mile radius of Upstate New York. His pigs are raised to be eaten. They are livestock."

My jaw dropped just enough to let her know I didn't know what to say.

I was at a loss for words, but the basis of her opinion was now in sharp focus. *Everything* she had ever had, from her American Girl dolls and her first pink tricycle to her brand new BMW and finally her Ivy League education, was the result of her father's pig farms. Not only was she raised thinking that pigs, highly-intelligent and sentient creatures, are *food*, but she is required to continue this myth for the rest of her life in order to vacation in the Caymans every year. She has to say these things in order to attend grad school and keep up with her friends in The Hamptons—and to, one day, have her dad pay for her perfect $175,000 wedding.

Pig blood ran through her family.

There was no way I would win, and there was no way I was going to continue the fight. She had *me* up against the ropes. On the brink of tears, feeling like I had been set up. Set up to be taken down by entitled omnivores.

Man cannot discover new oceans unless he
has the courage to lose sight of the shore.
—Andre Gide

During the fourth month of my veganism, I was sent on a business trip to Minnesota to conduct seminars for the construction company I was working for. I had never been to Minnesota and was a little shocked when I showed up in February and there was no snow. Arriving at the 1970s-style hotel conference center, I was immediately greeted by an ominous eight-foot-tall stuffed brown bear, advertising a local taxidermy business. And if memory serves correctly, the bear was standing on a bearskin rug. Next to the deceased and erected bear was a vendor table offering handmade wooden gun racks, boot racks, and coffee tables made out of massive tree trunks. I started to feel like perhaps this convention wasn't going to be all that vegan-friendly and that eating *might* be a challenge.

A traveling vegan faces challenges in procuring items that omnivores take for granted. Airports and airplanes offer almost only non-vegan and overprocessed food options. Too many times I've found myself falling back onto a box of french fries or into a bag of potato chips for comfort between the baby carrots and hummus I pretend to love. This Minnesota trip proved to be even more imposing.

Buffalo Wild Wings, Dairy Queen, KarmelKorn Shoppes, Old Country Buffet, Orange Julius, and T. G. I. Friday's are all headquartered in the Twin Cities of Minneapolis and St. Paul, and the predominantly German population brought over the Wiener schnitzel and wurst. Lots of wurst.

Midwesterners love meat. And the group I was traveling with were all infamous meat eaters and delighted to be in Minnesota, Spamtown USA.

Dinner plans were made for a local steakhouse, and "the guys" were already talking about what they would order and making jokes about "the probability of a vegan menu in a steakhouse," adding jibes about how much I was going to love my salad. Little did I know how right they would be.

Earlier that day, adjacent to the lobby, the hotel restaurant was alive with fur-lined denim jackets, leather pants, and cowboy boots. Everyone started their day waiting in line at the omelet station. They would choose their meat, vegetables, and cheese and watch as it was folded into three sizzling eggs that had just been freshly cracked, dropped into a quarter cup of sizzling oil, and scrambled with whole milk.

Meanwhile, I was once again finding myself eating a bowl of oatmeal with strawberries, trying to breathe in the seductive aroma of bacon and eggs. I had had a similar trip to New York City, where my two traveling companions ordered the "Lumberjack Special" while I ate a bowl of oatmeal, fruit, and home fries. I think limited vegan breakfast options while traveling may be why my love for potatoes started early on in my vegan journey.

It was during this same New York City trip that I watched a man standing beside a garbage can eating chicken wings, tearing the meat off and throwing the bare bone into the trash. This may have actually been the very first moment I started thinking to myself how odd it was that humans eat meat in the way he was eating meat off another animal's leg.

Carpooling to the steakhouse, I was still trying to be optimistic about finding vegan menu options. There would be *something*, right? The place was packed, so we waited forty-five minutes at the bar until the server finally seated us in a large horseshoe-shaped leather booth. She handed out menus and started taking our orders.

"I'll have the rib eye."

"I'll have the New York strip."

"I'll get the surf and turf."

"What do you have that I can get rare? I mean, how rare is legal in Minnesota?" They all laughed heartily, one of those movie laughs that keeps echoing and echoing until—dead silence. A record scratch. It was my turn.

"And you, hon?" The server asked as all eyes turned my way.

This was the moment they were waiting for. What does a vegan order at a steakhouse in Minnesota? This is the kind of moment books are written about (you're holding the proof). I had spent five full minutes scouring the menu, trying to extract meat and cheese from every item, to no avail. With the menu still open and all eyes fixed on me, I answered.

"Can I get your Cobb salad *without* bacon, egg, *or* bleu cheese?"

"Sure. Cobb salad. No meat. No egg. No cheese. Coming right up." She quickly jotted it down on her pad and whisked herself away. That was too easy.

"Great. And a basket of fries," I yelped across the busy dining room. Always had to order french fries, my inflatable life raft in a sea of good-for-you vegetables.

The server came back with the drink order, which was accompanied by a steamy loaf of bread. Everyone dove in, tore off a piece, and offered the basket to me. I looked at the bubbly, warm, beautiful gift and quickly noticed it had been brushed with melted butter and sprinkled with grated cheese. Of course. What's bread without butter and cheese? "No thanks," I said. I was still waiting on my french fries and meat-free, egg-free, cheese-free salad.

Years before I went vegan, I was on a business trip in Bloomington, Illinois. Driving the rental car from the Chicago airport, I kept passing "Culver's" restaurant locations. Under the logo on every sign, it read: "Home to the 'ButterBurger.'" During the half-day marketing retreat, I could hardly contain myself thinking about Culver's and anxiously waited for the client to announce it was lunchtime. It finally was.

"Where do you want to go?" Fran, my client contact, asked in her Midwestern accent. She was born and raised in Bloomington.

My eyes glazed over as if I were suddenly a zombie, and I replied in my best Homer Simpson voice, "Mmmm. Butter. Burger."

"You want to go to Culver's?" Fran asked, with a knowing smirk and an infectious Midwestern giggle. "I bet they don't have ButterBurgers in New York, do they?"

"No," I said, falling further in love with her voice—or maybe it was the fact that she had just used the words *butter* and *burger* together in a sentence, pressed right up against each other. The only way those two words were meant to be said.

"What is a ButterBurger anyway?" Oh, I was so innocent back then.

"A burger and bun, cooked in butter."

A ButterBurger is a burger that is cooked in butter, but to make it better, they also butter the bun and cook the bun in butter. Say that three times fast. Some Wisconsinites will tell you that a proper ButterBurger is when the ground meat is actually mixed with butter. For others, it's only a ButterBurger when the bun is toasted in butter and crowned with a pat of butter before it's served. There are probably even some purists out there who insist that the chef who cooks the burger must be slathered head to toe in butter. All lovers of a ButterBurger agree on one thing. There should be enough butter to drip off of the burger patty and pool into a puddle on your plate while you wolf down the half-pound patty.

We sped there as fast as we could. She was on a mission to show me what a ButterBurger was all about, and I was on a mission to be schooled.

It was only 11:30 a.m. The line for the drive-through was already five cars wide (and deep) as the busy uniformed employees ran bag after butter-stained bag of ButterBurgers out to the hungry Bloomingtonians. Fran and I found a corner booth, and I trusted her to place the order. Within ten very long minutes, our order was up. Fran brought the burgers back to our table with a huge, knowing smile on her face.

One bite of the hot ButterBurger, and I knew exactly what Midwest living tasted like. It tasted like butter—and what a heart attack must taste like.

Heart disease and stroke are, respectively, the first and third leading causes of death and also the major causes of disability in Illinois. In 2014, there were more than thirty thousand deaths in Illinois due to heart disease and over seven thousand deaths due to stroke. That's nearly forty thousand residents of Illinois who will never again enjoy a ButterBurger, which they shouldn't have in the first place.

Fast-forward a few years later: back at the Minnesota Steakhouse, the table was soon covered in every variety of steak mankind ever invented. And then even more steaks. Sizzling slabs of beef. A veritable jigsaw puzzle of flesh.

And my lone salad. Which was covered in bacon, egg, and bleu cheese.

"Excuse me?" Grabbing the server's attention before she flitted away, I said politely, "I ordered this *without* bacon, egg, or cheese; and this is covered in bacon, egg, *and* cheese." The server stared at me for a while as if to say, *oh, you were serious?*

Then she said, "Oh, you were serious?"

"Yeah, I'm vegan."

How do you know someone is vegan? Don't worry, they'll tell you, is how the joke goes. And I did. I wanted her to know that there was a legitimate reason I wouldn't eat the salad—as legitimate as being vegan gets.

She laughed and swept my meal away. As the others at the table cut and gnawed at their dinners like so many Flintstones, I was dipping my french fries in ketchup and admitting to myself that being vegan would all be worthwhile—and that I should not give in.

Do. Not. Give. In. It will get better.

The second attempt at my salad arrived, covered in bleu cheese and bacon. No egg. I cancelled my order and headed back to my hotel room to cry over a bag of potato chips.

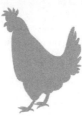

12

SURVIVAL MODE: ANYTHING YOU CAN EAT, I CAN EAT VEGAN

Extinction is the rule. Survival is the exception.
—Carl Sagan

I'll never forget, after first going vegan, how adamant I was to all my newfound vegan friends that there are simply "no good options" for eating vegan on-the-go and that this was clearly displayed in any vending machine in any bus or gas station in America—or in a Minnesota steakhouse. I was very sure of myself when I proclaimed that all on-the-go food you could buy while traveling simply does not exist for vegans. Sort of.

But, please note, you should not be eating vending machine food in the first place. To use a vending machine as an excuse when talking about available food is not the smartest strategy. You're immediately not taken seriously.

I can remember driving an hour and a half to and from work and stopping at the same gas station on the border of Pennsylvania and New York to buy coffee and a snack. The first few times I would stare, longingly, at the sausage breakfast sandwiches rotating under the hot lamps behind the grease-splattered glass and wondered why I couldn't eat *just one*. Bite into the outer croissant and feel the burn of butter as it ran down my chin. Licking the shiny fat residual off my fingers. Scraping the melted cheese from my teeth. Basking in the goodness that is cheap gas station rotisserie food.

Instead, I bought a banana.

And you know what? I was much better off. Since these early days, I've found many opportunities to satisfy any craving with something healthy (or unhealthy, since most potato chips are vegan, and potatoes still rule my life).

Within my first week of being vegan, I made this potato chip discovery. If potato chips are vegan, then I know I can always survive. I'll fill my trunk full of potato chips in case I'm ever stranded, and then I know I can still live happily ever after. If I ever find myself shipwrecked on a deserted island, I can always buy a bag of potato chips. From a deserted island vending machine.

When I found a popular brand of kettle chips at a rest stop outside of Pennsylvania, I was so excited. Digging my hand into the bag all the way home, I couldn't wait to share them with Jen. So I only ate half the bag. They were so tasty. And crunchy. And greasy. And life-sustaining. And, as Jen pointed out to me, since she actually reads labels: fried in lard.

Lard isn't vegan. It is one of those ingredients, like gelatin from horse hooves, that really makes me disgusted when I consider how humans have figured out a use for every part of the animal, and how we've made asinine claims that this is somehow good for the animals. Backing up a bit, animals are not food and shouldn't be considered a commodity—and frying potato chips in animal fat is just wrong. The newest yuppie culinary trend is duck fat french fries. Talk about ruining my favorite food by frying it in duck fat.

Lesson learned: read labels. Other lesson learned? Don't read labels while driving. Also, if you're reading a label, and there are words you can't pronounce, you're better off not eating it, especially with on-the-go food at gas stations or convenience stores.

To recap: Never eat anything you can't pronounce. Except quinoa. Always eat quinoa.

Meanwhile, there *are* fast-food, on-the-go vegan options out there, but it takes a well-seasoned vegan to point them out (please see page 171 for a comprehensive list of vegan fast-food options). Here, you do have to consider whether or not you're going vegan to improve your health, since a daily stop at In-N-Out for their fries and protein-style veggie wrap isn't going to necessarily loosen your belt. If your goal is to get healthy, I will refer you to a whole food plant-based diet. But, for now, let's stick to the vegan diet so we can all get through this together.

Every form of addiction is bad, no matter whether the narcotic be
alcohol, morphine, or idealism.
—*C. G. Jung*

Ah, cheese. That last step for vegetarians to make the full transition to a vegan diet. Let me go on record here as saying: It's not easy giving up cheese and dairy. They are addictive, literally. There is something called casomorphins that can be found in cheese. It is as strong as nicotine, just much tastier and amazing grilled into a sandwich or shmeered onto an everything bagel.

It takes ten pounds of cow's milk to make just one pound of cheese. As milk is turned into cheese, most of its water is removed, leaving behind pure casein, opiates, and the fabulous fat that gives it its texture. So, needless to say, concentrated dairy products like cheese are very high in fat, have especially high levels of opiates, and contain actual morphine.

To give you an idea of what this does to your body, here is an actual warning from The Center for Women's Healthcare (cfwhc.com), a healthcare website that explains the risks associated with morphine. I've edited it here for the cheese lover in all of us by replacing the word *morphine* with *cheese*:

Cheese can slow or stop your breathing. Never eat cheese in larger amounts, or for longer than a standard appetizer round.

You should not eat cheese if you have severe asthma or breathing problems, a blockage in your stomach or intestines, or a bowel obstruction called paralytic ileus.

Swallow cheese whole to avoid exposure to a potentially fatal dose.

Cheese may be habit-forming, even at regular doses. Never share cheese with another person, especially someone with a history of cheese abuse or addiction. Keep cheese in a place where others cannot get to it.

Tell your doctor if you are pregnant. Cheese may cause life-threatening withdrawal symptoms in a newborn.

Okay, so in all fairness, it's a very, very small dose of morphine in cheese; but if you eat a lot of cheese over the course of forty years like I did, it *can* be very addictive, and it *does* adversely affect your health. And cheese can be very appealing, especially when presented in pretty, edible packages.

I will never forget the day I discovered brie en croute before my veganism. Some innovative company created an off-the-shelf oversized hockey puck pastry filled with a delicious variety of brie flavors that I would fall in love with. Cut off the shrink wrap and bake for thirty minutes. Out of the oven comes a crusty bread filled with a gooey, pungent cheese. I would eat the whole wheel in one sitting. Servings per container = six.

Then I discovered how easy this was to make at home, thanks to the Pillsbury Dough Boy, and I was on my way to adding brie en croute as an appetizer to every dinner party from then on out. Brie, along with smoked Gouda from Vermont, English farmhouse cheddar, Gruyère, and Buffalo mozzarella were all a part of my usual culinary repertoire.

My fascination with cheese was only rivaled by my love for meat, and when I discovered you could actually *dip* meat into *cheese*, I was a goner. Fondue and elaborate cheese boards and banquet tables engulfed my life. Cheese was everywhere and everything to me for a long time.

So, how can you expect anyone to transition from this world of cheese to a world of "fake" cheeses made of God-knows-what? Let me be honest here, it wasn't easy at first, but plant-based chefs, food scientists, and very innovative companies have made it easier.

A *lot* easier. I can talk you down. Step away from the cheese wheel.

In just the last few years, delectable vegan cheese has taken on a life of its own. From organic, all-natural, traditionally prepared artisan options to American slices that taste just like American slices. Companies like Miyoko's Kitchen (based in California) have created gourmet cheeses that rival any of the finest European cheeses you'll ever taste, while industry leaders such as Follow Your Heart, Daiya, Field Roast, and VioLife have perfected the everyday cheeses, so much so that you could find yourself eating cheese every day.

Vegan cheese has arrived. Along with it, the number of nondairy milks has also expanded to such an extent that there is no longer any good reason to consume cow's milk in any form ever again. Unless, of course, you're a baby cow.

There are nut milks (almond, cashew), soy milk, hemp milk, oat milk, and even pea milk. While pea milk doesn't sound at all appetizing, it's surprisingly the best of the bunch. Maybe not so surprising when you remember that it's spelled P-E-A (I'll openly admit that pee milk would be bad; and depending on whose pee, it may not even be vegan). Each of the actual vegan milks is fortified with more calcium, Vitamin D, and essential nutrients than the traditional dairy milks. For the record, some naysayers about nondairy milk might throw around statistics about almond milk contributing to the California drought (it's nothing compared to the number of cows in that state) or almond milk as being somehow less than trustworthy since it actually contains only 2 percent almonds. Remind these folks that every cup of coffee contains 2 percent coffee and 98 percent water.

Cow's milk is naturally loaded with hormones that are best suited to make little cows into big cows. Quickly. Giving that same milk to a human, especially a human baby, is overkill. Humans simply don't need the mix of nutrients that cow's milk provides. Even "hormone-free" cow's milk contains nearly sixty hormones, just not *artificially added* hormones. Cow's milk contains estrogen and is a known cause of breast, ovarian, and uterine cancers. All cows that produce milk are pregnant, even the ones labeled grass-fed or free-range or organic.

So, why are humans the only animals who drink the milk of another species, and why do we even continue to drink milk as adults? And why don't people make these seemingly simple connections whenever they are choosing to purchase other milks available on the market—goat, sheep, or even buffalo milk? Any of these are as useful and natural to human health as cat's milk or giraffe's milk.

How did this happen?

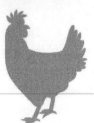

13

THE HISTORY OF MILK, EGGS, AND THE WORLD

*The human body has no more need for cows' milk
than it does for dogs' milk, horses' milk, or giraffes' milk.*
—*Michael Klaper, MD.*

I imagine the discovery of cow's milk for humans went something like this.

The year is 10,000 BC, in an alternate reality, General Nakhtmin of the Seventh Egyptian Army enters the temple of Queen Nakhtubasterau. She is looking forlorn.

"My Queen, what is it that I can bring to you to satisfy your longing?" Nakhtmin asked, removing his helmet as any good general would do in the presence of royalty, or if it didn't fit under a doorway, or he didn't want to get "helmet head."

"General, Princess Reputnebty has been weaned. She is now three-renpets of age and one short cubit tall and is requesting *milk*. Milk that I can no longer provide to her." She covered her face with her hands in shame, peeking through her fingers at Nakhtmin to make sure he was still listening.

"My Queen," General Nakhtmin offered. "I cannot bear to see you this way. I shall search all of Egypt, until I find a suitable replacement for milk for Princess Reputnebty. This, my majesty, shall be my only reason to live. This, and figuring out how the pyramids were made. It's pretty incredible, actually. They're so large."

And so, General Nakhtmin and his army set out that night on a quest to find milk for Princess Reputnebty. They sandaled past the pyramids, stopping in wonderment, and a quick selfie, until they came upon a sand snake, slithering across the sand (hence the name).

"Oh, great serpent, as you are the symbol of fertility, I look to you to provide milk for the Queen's youngest." General Nakhtmin ordered one of his minions to capture the snake and, upon squeezing it, licking it, and examining it lengthwise and widthwise, could not find nipples. He chucked the snake aside and carried on.

As they approached the Sphinx, General Nakhtmin stared upon it, and inspiration dawned on him.

I need a very large cat, he thought.

The General peered under the front porch (few people know that the Sphinx has a very nice front porch) and spied a stray cat—nursing her young. Removing the tiny, hungry kittens with a flick of his massive fingers, he was disappointed to discover that her nipples were too small for a human mouth to properly latch onto. So, he moved along.

"Snakes have no nipples. Cat nipples are too small to get a solid latch. I must find an animal precisely the right size who is lactating, in order to provide the Princess with milk," he mused.

Then, high upon a sand dune, he spotted a lactating camel. Interesting sidebar: some of the very first milk consumed by humans was, in fact, camel milk. Now, back to our story. The general made his way under the camel and found that he couldn't easily reach the teats. Egyptians were fairly short back then.

"If I cannot reach, the Princess surely can't," he said to himself, now growing more impatient.

Frustrated and tired, he continued farther into the fields until he spotted a spotted cow, her teats dripping with milk. He approached the beast.

"This cow," General Nakhtmin proclaimed, holding his hand up to God Ra-Horakhty, "is in obvious pain and discomfort and needs to be milked to provide her relief. This is the cow that shall provide milk for the Queen and Princess Reputnebty! And, from now on, I proclaim that all cows throughout the kingdom shall be corralled for their precious gift of milk. My work here is done."

General Nakhtmin's army brought the cow over field and sand back to the palace of the Queen and presented her with a bow. As in, they bowed down, not with a bow, like a gift.

"Your highness, fetch little Princess Reputnebty and place her gently under this lactating cow, for *she* shall nourish upon the teat as if she, herself, were a young calf."

Delighted, the Queen fetched the princess and placed the young child under the cow, smiling as the hungry girl attempted to latch on and was eventually trampled.

It took another hundred years before Egyptians finally figured out how to actually *milk* the cows and another 12,214 years before humans were able to wean themselves from cow's milk for good and fully understand that milk doesn't actually do a body good.

> *"Animals are not products. Life doesn't have a price."*
> *—Anonymous*

Contrary to what you've been told since you were a wee one, milk is not good for you. In fact, the dairy industry has been lying to us for years. Overproduction of milk following the Second World War started a focused effort to sell more milk. To do so, the dairy industry began fabricating and advertising the benefits of milk and telling all of us that milk makes strong bones.

The exact opposite is true. According to the Physicians Committee for Responsible Medicine (PCRM) and Dr. Greger from NutritonFacts.org, milk leaches calcium from bones. Decades of consuming milk in an effort to get stronger actually makes us weaker. There is a reason why your grandmother's hip keeps breaking with simple falls; her bones have become brittle.

> *Cruelty might be very human, and it might*
> *be cultural, but it's not acceptable.*
> *—Jodi Foster*

I was sitting in my office one day when a coworker knocked on the door. She took the seat across from me and had a look of "I'm going to ask you a question about being vegan," and I was right.

Jane (her real name is Janet, but she didn't want me to use her real name in this book) is one of those people who has always circled around the subject of becoming vegan, and she's still a contender for transitioning to veganism full-time. However, she is also someone who is continually misfed information about the health benefits, and ethics, of certain foods that vegans choose not to eat.

"Can I ask you a question?" she asked, which means she had already answered that question on her own.

"Sure," I said, taking a bite of my Macro Mama's Spicy Peanut Lime Noodles. This particular Asian-inspired dish is so popular at the Ithaca Farmer's Market and at specialty grocers in the region that it has been a contender for the "Official Food of Ithaca" for years. It's like crack. Peanutty, noodly crack.

"What's wrong with milk? You don't *have to kill* the cows to get their milk," she lamented. "Right?"

Oh, Jane (Janet). Come here. You need a vegan hug.

Of course she's right. *Technically*, you don't. Milking a cow really could be a rather harmless and benign process. But, of course, milking a cow is not something humans are actually meant to do. So I answered her question for her, trying my hardest not to step up on the soapbox I kept under my desk for these occasions.

"Technically, you don't," I started, as I carefully stepped up onto my soapbox that I was scooting out from under my desk. "But what you *have* to realize about the dairy industry is that it's *actually* the *meat* industry. There is more rape, torture, and slaughter that goes into one glass of milk than you'd find in an entire steak."

I began centering myself on my box, hoping others in the hall were listening in.

"You see, in order for cows to actually *give* milk, they need to be *lactating*, and in order for them to be lactating, they need to become pregnant and *give birth*. Now, to start this process, most dairy cows are artificially inseminated by a farmer who inserts his entire arm up a cow's anus to properly position her uterus in order to ensure a precise injection of the bull's semen. Once pregnant, like humans, the cow waits nine months to give birth to her young. These newborn offspring are ripped away from the mother cow so *they* don't take the milk that is being produced for them but that ends up being extracted for *your* consumption."

I started to hold up one hand like a preacher at Hyde Park. I had the floor, and I wasn't going to let this one get away.

"*If* the newborn calf is female, she is likely raised to live the same life as her mother. Bred to become impregnated over and over again so she will spend her lifetime lactating. A lifetime of rape, birth, and servitude. If this offspring is *male* . . ." I closed my eyes and slowly shook my head in disbelief; I was pouring as much drama into this performance as I ever have. "If this offspring is male, he is moved into a small plastic box, which will prevent him from moving around and growing muscle, and he will be killed within a few months of birth to become veal. *This* is your dairy industry."

Her eyes were beginning to glaze over. I knew I had her at this point. Besides, I had locked my office door from the inside.

"These dairy cows are *also* pumped full of hormones to force their bodies to produce up to three times as much milk as they naturally produce, and their bodies are subjected to ongoing and uncomfortable constant milking, which causes sores and pus discharge. Once they're no longer able to be impregnated or are too old and worn out to lactate, they are slaughtered for meat.

"This is happening over *nine million times per day* in the United States alone. All to produce an *unhealthy* product that humans *shouldn't* be consuming in the first place. Milk from cows is for baby cows. In fact, we've all been lied to for decades about the health advantages of drinking milk. You know how your grandma has fallen and 'she can't get up'? Well, that's because her bones have been weakened by all the dairy she's been consuming since the war. Grandma's not getting up."

I heard rousing applause in my head. And nothing from Jane (Janet). She stood up and slinked out of my office with a very quiet, "M'kay, thanks."

A week later she asked the exact same question. About eggs.

I was eating in a Chinese restaurant downtown.
There was a dish called Mother and Child Reunion.
It's chicken and eggs. And I said, I gotta use that one.
—*Paul Simon*

Confession time. I loved eggs. I loved all 101 ways to prepare eggs. Fried. Over easy, Sunny side up. Scrambled. Poached. Soft boiled. Hard boiled. You name it, I ate it. I loved cooking with eggs, cracking them on the edge of the bowl with one hand and adding them to my baked goods, and I even loved blowing them. Every Easter, we would poke a small pinhole in one end of the egg and a slightly larger pinhole in the other, and then blow out the contents to create a hollow egg. Blowing eggs gave me an eggasm. Eggs were as essential to my breakfast as toast and sausage, and giving them up was actually harder to do than cheese.

But I did. Overnight.

Woke up vegan and looked around our little kitchen and wondered what vegans ate for breakfast. Checked the refrigerator. Nothing. Checked the pantry. Nothing. Other than home fries and toast, everything else I loved was off the table. And there is no way you will ever convince me that a green smoothie is breakfast; a breakfast needs to be hot meal, a blue-plate special.

"Two poached eggs, whole wheat toast, sausage, home fries, chocolate milk, and a cup of black coffee," I said to Chris, our server, every morning at my Rotary International breakfast meeting.

Our meetings were held at the Royal Court Restaurant. A hotel restaurant with more dark wood paneling than should be legal and fake oil paintings of bridges and horses. If I'm not mistaken, the bar was made out of old carriage wheels. You get the picture.

I would eat here every morning for years, ordering the same exact thing. Or, I'd eat at the nearby State Diner, still ordering the same thing. This was my breakfast, and I was taking that to the grave, or so I thought. And now, this first morning vegan, I couldn't have my usual, and possibly never again if I planned on not losing The Bet.

There is a famous tiny restaurant in Oswego, New York, called Wade's. Wade, a six-foot-tall wrinkled man, who probably weighed ninety pounds, would stand hunched over his greasy stainless steel stovetop and crack eggs with one hand and then toss the shells behind him, underhanded, so they would smash under the counter right where you were sitting. He probably went through a thousand eggs each morning, making every variation of egg imaginable. In fact, I don't remember ever eating anything *but* eggs at Wade's.

Three eggs over easy, whole wheat toast, and a cup of black coffee. Now that was a breakfast, and at Wade's it probably cost $2.75.

Now here I was, staring down the barrel of an eggless breakfast future.

I asked my vegan friends what they ate for breakfast, and it was not the least bit surprising to hear how they "enjoyed" (who really enjoys this?) oatmeal with fresh fruit or some variation of a kale smoothie. One delusional vegan told me she ate half a watermelon, which was "as satisfying as the best cheese omelet [she'd] ever eaten."

Oh my God, she was lying. There was no way this was true. Reflecting back, I still think this ranks among the highest for "ridiculous things vegans have ever said to me."

Still, there I was, eggless. No starting point for a hot breakfast. The first few weeks, I actually *did* eat fruit. Stood around the kitchen like an ape. Crunching on an apple or gnawing on a banana. Climbing the walls in search of a mango. This was not sustainable. *Man need breakfast.*

I pounded my chest. Probably more to knock some of the accumulated plaque off my arteries than anything else.

And then a couple of things happened. First, I learned how to make a tofu scramble (recipe at the end of this book) that eventually rivaled any egg recipe I used to eat. Simple and delicious, and packed with protein, fiber, and zero cholesterol. Second, a popular vegan company came out with a vegan egg that is pretty much a clone for traditional eggs, with no chicken intervention.

The VeganEgg from Follow Your Heart is a revolutionary product that comes in a powder or liquid form and is the right blend of ingredients that, when whisked, becomes a very convincing egg "batter." You can French toast it, use it as an ingredient in baked goods, turn it into an omelet, or simply scramble it. Pour the VeganEgg onto a hot, oiled surface, and in a few minutes, you're eating "eggs."

The taste and texture is as close to a chicken's egg as you'll find anywhere. When this product first came out, it sold out in nearly every retail setting instantly, which is probably why they now offer it in five-pound buckets.

If you can't find this product near you, there are ways to make your own variation using chickpea flour, water, and the right spices. Specifically, Black Himalayan Crystal Salt, or Kala Namak. This unique spice has a sulfuric taste and, when added to a chickpea flour omelet or a tofu scramble, mimics the smell and taste of an egg.

Breakfast was back. Scrambled eggs with green peppers and onions, vegan sausage, home fries, toast, vegan chocolate milk, and black coffee.

And no one had to die.

Animals are not ingredients.
—Barbara Thompson

Jane (Janet) came back into my office and sat down. She was playing with the stapler on the edge of my desk when she timidly asked, "So, what's wrong with eating eggs? You don't have to *kill* chickens to get their eggs."

Taking a deep breath, I pushed my soapbox onto the spot on the floor I marked with tape. I always waited patiently for these moments, and Jane (Janet) was wonderful to have around.

"Well," I said, straightening the suit jacket I wasn't wearing, "Eggs are not unlike the chicken's monthly 'period.' Their unfertilized egg drops down and is expelled from their bodies. These unfertilized eggs, in the wild, become a protein source for the birds and other animals who may stumble upon them. If *that* isn't enough to turn you off from eating eggs," I continued, "you should know that the egg industry kills upward of 250 thousand male chicks daily by tossing them into a grinder. Alive. This is called 'culling.' Male chicks are useless in the industry, since they can't lay eggs. Don't even get me started on backyard hens."

I made that last statement with a "talk to the hand" gesture and stepped down.

"One more thing. When a hen gets old, she starts producing eggs *without* shells. Imagine that the next time you crack an egg in the morning. Of course, most hens are slaughtered before the farmer has to start scraping that mess off the floor of his coop."

Backing off my soapbox, I had said all I needed to say about eggs. This was a much shorter performance, as I had a meeting that would start in five minutes.

Jane (Janet) thanked me and crossed the hall back to her office. For the record, she's still not vegan. Maybe I need a bigger soapbox.

In June of 2016, United Egg Producers surprised us all with an announcement that changed how egg production is perceived forever. In what counts as huge news in the animal welfare world, the industry group, which represents the hatcheries that produce 95 percent of all eggs in the United States, announced that it would end the culling of millions of male chicks by 2020, or as soon as they find that it is "economically feasible." An alternative that is "commercially available," according to the Humane League, is called in-ovo sexing. It actually identifies the gender of a future chick inside a fertilized egg.

The technology, developed in Germany and the Netherlands, will mean that male chicks will never be born—or ground or gassed or suffocated, the kill methods some hatcheries employ. Even with this advancement, the question is still begged: at what point are these fertilized eggs sentient? Other alternatives are also being explored, including one that would turn male chick eggs a different color from those of females.

Of course, there are two views of this solution.

"Their sisters are still going to be slaughtered, and they're going to spend eighteen months in a cage where they can never spread their wings," Paul Shapiro, vice president of farm animal protection at the Humane Society of the United States, said. "Eighteen months of unmitigated misery is far worse than what happens to these male chicks."

Healthy is merely the slowest rate at which one can die.
—Unknown

One of the more frequent comments about a vegan diet made by omnivores regards soy, the little green bean that has been causing controversy.

Meat eaters are often embarrassed to admit the real reason they shy away from soy-based meat substitutes, including tofu. I've been pulled aside at countless cookouts and plenty of potlucks and asked, privately, if eating tofu would slowly make its consumer more . . . effeminate? Will the so-called "toxic levels of estrogen" they've heard so much about that are found in soy somehow lessen their manliness?

"I heard, you know, that I'll get man boobs or something," a friend whispered to me as he drank his Labatt's beer and tried not to enjoy the barbecued grilled tofu po'boy I had brought to the backyard barbecue.

"You already have man boobs, Bob," I whispered back.

"You're funny. I'm being serious."

"So am I."

Since I'm actually a nice guy, I explained to him the true dangers of soy and tofu in detail. Tofu is derived from soy, the edamame bean, and is an excellent source of protein, fiber, and various amino acids, with low levels of fat and sugar. It's also a good source of minerals such as calcium, iron, magnesium, phosphorus, potassium, sodium, zinc, copper, and manganese. But it's mostly popular because it's a very versatile ingredient in many dishes. Tofu originated in the Han Dynasty in China some two thousand years ago, which is why it's been a main ingredient in so many Asian dishes. But, be warned, some believe it *can* be dangerous for some men.

"So, will eating it turn me into a woman?"

As most meat eaters will tell you, since they are always so well informed, there are certain risks associated with eating too much soy (tofu). From personal experience, I know that any time I tell someone I eat tofu, they suddenly turn into nutritionists who warn me against its adverse health consequences. But what they often overlook, and what they are actually referring to, is a little-known side effect of *men* eating too much tofu:

"*Growavaginaitis.*"

"Grow a what?" he asked, spitting out the tofu and taking a long, manly gulp of his beer.

"You heard me. Forget about your man boobs, you've got bigger things to worry about. Down. There."

I had his attention.

"Supposedly, tofu acts like a super-charged estrogen. When men eat too much of it, well, first they form breasts—and you're already on your way to having a nice rack—but soon after, you'll begin to grow a vagina."

"You're full of it."

"Tofu?" I asked, smirking, offering him another serving of barbecue tofu, which he vehemently refused.

Of course, there are risks and side effects associated with everything we eat, so why should soy be any different? Leading experts will recommend no more than three to four servings *per day*. But, more important, why should meat eaters care so much about soy?

They care because soy is the biggest threat to big meat.

I'll say that again, because it's actually pretty clever and would make an excellent T-shirt: *Soy is the biggest threat to big meat.*

The meat industry doesn't want viable, versatile, and healthier alternative protein sources to exist. Once we all discover new nutrient-rich sources of protein (and regular sources of B12), it's over. The meat, dairy, and egg industries will feel the pinch and eventually collapse. These healthier replacements are already having an impact on these industries, and it's not going to slow down or reverse. Soy is so readily available, proven healthy, and extremely versatile that it can be used in place of virtually any meat.

From silken to firm, tofu is a white block of goodness that takes on whatever personality you ask of it; and, when grilled, baked, scrambled, or cooked to perfection, it adds a delicious bite to any dish.

As much as omnivores have had it drilled into them that meat *isn't* bad for them and that they need milk for calcium and eggs for protein, they are also being fed half-truths about soy. Think about it; if there were an alternative food for everything meat (and dairy), the only reason people would continue to eat those foods would be that they hate animals.

They would be killing and eating animals for absolutely no reason. Sort of like the way things are today, but with no real excuses.

Is there a limit to how much soy you should consume? And what about the quality? Of course there is a limit to how much of anything you should consume, even water. Dr. Michael Greger, of NutritionFacts. org, recommends no more than three to five servings of tofu per day, and you should make sure it's organic and non-GMO. That's a lot of soy per day. You may also want to remind your soy-fearing omnivore friends that the soy that is *not* fit for human consumption is being fed to livestock—to *their* food. So, it actually turns out they're the ones who are eating the *bad* soy.

Dr. Greger also reports that soy has some decidedly incredible health advantages you can't find in other foods. Studies have repeatedly found that women who eat lots of soy appear to have a lower risk of getting breast cancer and a better risk of surviving breast cancer than those who don't.

The dairy industry doesn't want you to know that, either. Their pitchmen say soy has estrogen, which promotes breast cancer. But that's wrong. Soy contains phytoestrogens, chemicals that are similar enough to estrogen to bind to estrogen receptors in tumors, but different enough not to promote tumor growth. In fact, the evidence suggests that phytoestrogens block the more dangerous estrogen, which is why countries with high soy consumption have less, not more, breast cancer than countries with low soy consumption.

So, grab a firm brick of tofu and grill it, fry it, bake it, blend it, scramble it, slice it, press it, and enjoy it!

Be a man about it.

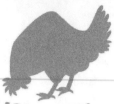

14

POOP AND OTHER BODILY FUNCTIONS VEGANS GO ON ABOUT

Everybody looks at their poop.
—Oprah Winfrey

A book about veganism wouldn't be complete without a chapter on poop. In fact, name one piece of classic literature that wouldn't benefit from a chapter about the one thing everyone (hopefully) does on a daily basis—and, if you're vegan, you may do as many as five times per day.

The word *poop* comes from the onomatopoeia *poupen* or *popen*, which originally meant "fart." The more you know. *Poop* came into its current meaning around 1900—and every person poops.

Historians poop.

All famous writers poop.

Politicians poop.

Actors poop, too.

Vegans poop more, and vegan actors might poop the most.

Since a plant-based diet is naturally high in fiber, which keeps your plumbing nice and operational, you're going to poop more. Eliminate dairy. And eliminate better, and more often.

I can't tell you the number of parents I know who have called off playdates because their little ones are painfully constipated, sitting on the potty for hours, crying. In fact, we have vegan friends who actually have nonvegan kids suffering from chronic constipation that is directly connected to their diet and dairy intake.

A diet high in cheese and other low-fiber/high-fat foods such as eggs and meat can slow down your digestion and cause constipation. If you want to poop, go vegan. Even if you don't want to poop, go vegan. There are so many alternatives to dairy products that there is no reason ever to consume dairy again, and the earlier you can start your kids eating these vegan versions, the better.

When you first go vegan, your bowel regularity will be more obvious as your body is getting rid of the waste leftover from the meat, cheese, and milk and getting accustomed to an increased amount of fresh, colon-cleansing foods in your diet. You're also going to find that your bathroom activity is easier and more pleasant, inasmuch as pooping would ever be considered "pleasant."

Bring an iPad. Or this book. You're going to be needing it as many as five times a day. (After a few weeks, this may even out and you may only go twice a day.)

We've had meat-eating friends over to our house for weekend visits, and they kindly agree to dine all-vegan while staying with us. Whether we are going out, dragging them to Friday Dinner, or cooking at home, we like to impress them with the variety and tastiness of vegan cuisine.

And, inevitably, by Sunday night, we are all talking about the poop they are experiencing.

Everybody poops. Everyone from George Clooney to the Queen of England. Chances are they've probably pooped at the same time, although most likely not in the same place.

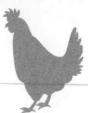

15

POTATOES:
THE OTHER WHITE MEAT

Every single diet I ever fell off of was because
of potatoes and gravy of some sort.
—Dolly Parton

I love potatoes. Let's face it: if I could, I would date a potato. I love them that much. Over time, I would really get to know the potato. We'd boat in Central Park. Go sightseeing in Atlantic City. Eventually, we'd fly out to meet her parents in Idaho.

I would let her know that I find her very appealing and then, while brushing the dirt off her skin, let her know I think she is beyond spectacular and not just a "common" tater. One day, I would look her in her eye and ask her to be my wife. We'd invite the Russets and the Kennebecs. Our wedding color theme would be red, white, and yellow, and we'd all get really smashed at the reception. But not on potato vodka; that would be cannibalism. We'd eventually move into a small apartment in the city and buy a place to "get away from it all" in Spud, Florida. And since we talked about it in advance, we'd one day have three little tots running around—and, eventually, I would eat her.

Because she is a potato, and I love her that much.

One of the crutches of the vegan diet for me has been the potato; in any form. Starting with the simple potato chip: kettle cooked. And expanding into mashed, hasslebacked, baked, roasted, saladed, shredded, hashbrowned, and finally: French fried.

When Jen and I honeymooned in London and Paris, we were a year and a half vegan and on a quest to dine in every vegan restaurant those two cities had to offer. Where we stayed in London was a half a block from a Whole Foods Market that, at that time, happened to have a nice vegan restaurant on the second floor. We were there every day. We also visited the famous Mildred's, Tibits, Wild Food Cafe, and Woodland's while jaunting around The Big Smoke. You'll find all the major cities of the world now boast an unbelievable array of vegan eateries, and in fact Taiwan, Singapore, Poland, and even Canada boast city centers rated in the Top Ten for their incredible vegan options.

It was while at VeganX, a small specialty shop off King's Cross Station outside of London, that we first got our taste of VioLife cheese. This Greek company has raised the bar unbelievably high for other vegan cheese companies to follow. When we were there, it wasn't yet available stateside. We purchased two packages of their sliced cheese and ate them rolled and plain on the sidewalk outside the shop.

Then we went back in and purchased two more, because we're Americans.

It was that good. It smelled and tasted like real dairy cheese, and the texture was perfect. Had we not visited London that year, I don't know if we would have ever discovered VioLife, a company I keep in touch with to this day, as they ship me products to sample on a regular basis.

Since Jen attended high school in London, she was the perfect tour guide for a full week of touring The Swinging City, after which we took the high-speed rail to Paris. The city of love.

I fell in love in, and with, Paris.

Since this was my first time in France's capital city, I skillfully prepared a list of all the required vegan restaurants and shops we needed to visit. One shop, which was less than a mile from our hotel, took us straight through the heart of the Parisian red light district. In case you're wondering, turns out Parisian hookers dress exactly as you would expect.

At one point a prostitute thought Jen was working her side of the street and accosted her, in French. While we had no idea what she was saying, her body language told the complete story, and Jen replied politely in French, "Sorry, I don't understand. I don't speak French."

We hoped that answered any of her questions, and we hurried along.

The little vegan shop we visited sold all the European versions of vegan foods we couldn't get in the United States; it also sold VioLife. So we bought some. And ate it. Walking back to the hotel, I couldn't help but notice an English-language spray-painted message written on a classic French doorway a few blocks away: "Go Vegan."

Then, as clichéd as a black beret and a black-and-white striped sweater, we ordered *pommes frites* at every restaurant in Paris. Sitting under the lights of the Eiffel Tower with my new wife, my heart fluttering and skipping a beat as I looked longingly . . . at a fried pile of thinly-sliced potatoes. . . my love for potatoes officially became international.

During Vegetarian Summerfest, the annual vegan event held in Johnstown, Pennsylvania, we got to see the infamous Dr. John McDougall speak at a packed auditorium right after the release of his book *The Starch Solution: Eat the Foods You Love, Regain Your Health, and Lose the Weight for Good!* He lit up the stage, dispelling the myths that starch and carbs lead to weight gain and waxed poetic about the potato.

He had me at *potato.*

"The more rice, corn, potatoes, sweet potatoes, and beans we eat, the trimmer, more energetic, and healthier we become," he said as he paced the massive stage in front of a thousand captive vegans. "Throughout civilization and around the world, six foods have provided our primary fuel: barley, corn, millet, potatoes, rice, and wheat."

I hung onto his every word. Well, mostly one word. He kept mentioning *potato.* This was the moment I was waiting for as a new vegan. Someone was finally going out on a limb and telling me I could live off of potatoes. Every meal could be potatoes. I was about to become validated. An excellent source of vitamin C with fantastic fiber and incredible iron, this low calorie, no cholesterol, low-in-fat root vegetable would be my everything.

He kept talking, and all I kept hearing was, "Potatoes. Potatoes. Potatoes. Potatoes."

After the talk, we rushed to meet Dr. McDougall offstage. My heart was fluttering with affection for this man as I nudged my way to the front of the line to greet him, pushing smaller, puny vegans aside. I finally made it up and asked, "So, you're saying I can live a long and healthy vegan life eating french fries?"

To which he replied: "No. No fried foods."

Heartbroken. I will never forgive John McDougall.

How healthy you are as a vegan is entirely up to you. If you're entering veganism from a health perspective, you may want to avoid all processed foods, fried foods, oil, sugar, and salt. But what fun is that?

It was at this same Summerfest that I met Chef AJ, a leading vegan chef and cookbook author. Her book *Unprocessed: How to Achieve Vibrant Health and Your Ideal Weight* features tips and recipes on living an unprocessed and healthy life by incorporating more fresh fruits and vegetables in your diet in ways that are easy, delicious, and fun. She is an outspoken and dynamic personality committed to great health through plant-based eating.

I met her at a book signing table and told her of my addiction to potatoes. I was hoping she would tell me I could continue eating french fries. I approached her as she looked up from signing a page.

"My name is Eric, and I'm a potatoholic."

"Hi, Eric."

I went on to tell her about my first six months as a vegan and how skeptical I had been in the beginning. I told her how I went vegan overnight on a bet. How I never really ate vegetables growing up. And I confessed to her that I was surviving off of french fries and knew that I probably needed to cut back. At that point, I was up to a pack a day.

AJ gave me a grin and said she was so convinced I could give them up that she inscribed the title page of her book with: *Dear Eric, I bet you can give up french fries for 30 days! Love Chef AJ."

Great, just what I needed. Another bet.

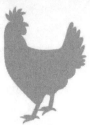

16

ABCs OF VEGANS

My whole life is waiting for the questions to which I have prepared
answers.
—*Tom Stoppard*

Just six months into being vegan, we were coaxed into attending Vegetarian Summerfest by a table full of vegans at Friday Dinner. This five-day vegan event, hosted by the North American Vegetarian Society, attracts thousands of hardcore vegans to a very remote part of Johnstown, Pennsylvania. A cult gathering in a remote part of Pennsylvania?

Remind me again, is KoolAid vegan, and why would I ever want to attend this event?

"Yeah, I don't think I'd like it," I said to Mike, a lawyer, author, friend, and vegan. He and his wife, Sherry, are both respected Cornell professors and have published countless blog posts, white papers, and books on veganism. Sherry's book *Mind if I Order the Cheeseburger?* goes into incredible depth answering, in perfect and precise detail, all the questions vegans are asked. The two of them are ardent animal rights advocates and outspoken protectors of all living creatures, and we remain good friends to this day.

Back in 2011, my first year being vegan, the fast casual restaurant Chipotle came out with a short film titled *Back to the Start* that went on to win an Academy Award. Set to the song "The Scientist," originally recorded by Coldplay and covered by Willie Nelson, the film beautifully portrays factory farming. It makes the viewer believe that Chipotle cared more about the pigs they raised and slaughtered than other fast food and fast casual restaurants.

Jen and I were sitting down to eat our vegan burrito bowls at Chipotle just as Sherry was leaving with her own vegan to-go order.

"Did you see that amazing Chipotle film showing how much better the conditions and treatment are for Chipotle's livestock?" I asked her, not expecting the answer I got.

"They're still killed in the end," Sherry said.

I was somewhat taken aback by her candor. It was still early days into my veganism. I had to stop to process exactly what she was saying from an animal rights perspective, as opposed to the perspective of an average consumer toward whom the animated short was obviously targeted.

Does the treatment of farm animals leading up to their death actually make a difference to the farm animals? It took me another year to finally understand exactly where she was coming from. But, before that epiphany, there was my first exposure to Summerfest.

"Why wouldn't you like Summerfest?" Mike asked, lowering a hot spoonful of butternut squash soup from his mouth.

"It sounds terrifying. I'm not really a big fan of hippies. Or the outdoors. Or vegans, to be honest." The room went quiet. "Except all of you," I quickly chuckled, darting my eyes around to see if I survived that comment.

Vegetarian Summerfest did sound terrifying at the time. I wasn't sure I wanted to be one of *them*. I certainly didn't want to spend five days *with* them. I was as skeptical and as reluctant as I ever would be. In the back of my mind, I knew I wasn't going to become one of these people. I was just passing by. Trying this out. Seeing where it would lead. I had no intention of unpacking my luggage and checking into Hotel Vegan.

Crazy Hotel Vegan.

Plus, Summerfest didn't even take place at a hotel or fancy convention center. It was a college campus, and you had to stay in single-bed dorm rooms with no air conditioning. There is only one thing worse than a hippy, and that's a hippy who smells bad.

I was not going to like Summerfest.

The six-hour drive was going to be a waste of time.

I was terrified.

To be safe, I made sure I packed my magic black vegan shirt.

It ended up not being terrifying at all, and there were very few hippies and only one guitar sing-along (that I witnessed). Go figure.

As a new vegan, it was actually refreshing knowing that everyone present was on the same page. Intelligent people were gathered together on what ended up being a beautiful campus, sharing ideas and experiences and learning from some of the industry's top thought leaders. Also, the endless vegan food was an undeniable perk. If you wonder how many vegans are in it for the bean sprouts and kale chips, just try standing in line at the pizza bar at Summerfest. They can't *make* vegan pizza fast enough to keep the vegans at bay.

The five days at Summerfest featured educational sessions, keynote speakers, cooking demos, and more vegans than you'd ever expect to see in one place in your life. It was here that I met Kristin Lajeunesse of *Will Travel for Vegan Food*, vegan superathlete Rich Roll, vegan chef and cheese queen Miyoko Schinner, and vegan pastry chef Fran Costigan.

I also got to meet Dr. Milton Mills and learned from his fascinating talk on why he believes humans are inherently herbivores. Not omnivores, but rather plant-munching herbivorous grazers. Milton demonstrated how a three-hundred-pound lion can eat over fifty-seven thousand calories per meal and then not eat again for seven to ten days. On the other hand, herbivores foraging for whole plant foods can't consume enough calories at one time to make it through just twenty-four hours and so must eat multiple times a day. Humans rarely eat raw meat, and our teeth are not equipped to tear uncooked flesh from a bone. We can eat apples rather easily, however.

Add to this the digestive tract of a lion as compared to a human. The lion's small intestine is just five feet long, while a human small intestine is roughly twenty feet long. This longer digestive system provides for numerous "pockets" where meat can get stopped and stuck, which may cause major health issues. This same meat passes quickly through a lion. Humans are not lions, and our bodies thrive on whole foods like fruits, vegetables, and whole grains.

Most important, it was during this Summerfest that I was privileged to see, live, for the very first time, what would end up being one of Dr. Michael Greger's most important, and most watched, talks of all time. *Uprooting the Leading Causes of Death* is a fifty-five-minute video that anyone who has ever considering going vegan for their health needs to watch. To date, it has been viewed over two million times on YouTube. I'll forgive you if you decide to dog ear (or, since that's not a vegan term, bookmark) this page right now to watch it. I'll just wait for you here.

Well, did you watch it? Pretty incredible isn't it?

Now, back to my story.

In addition to meeting amazing chefs, doctors, authors, filmmakers, and athletes at Summerfest, I got to make many new friends, with whom I stay in touch today. With endless introductions over meals, at breakout sessions, and even during karaoke, this event made me recognize the true meaning of being vegan and its positive impact on my health and the planet.

Summerfest ended up being the on-ramp to the highway of my veganism.

Probably the most enlightening part of Summerfest was discovering the wide array of vegans that exist in the world. Vegans frequently fall into certain cliques and categories, but what I found out at Summerfest is that we are all *very* different. So, I will now submit the alphabetical, tear-out (not literally, although you're welcome to, since you own the book) reference guide to "The ABCs of Being Vegan":

Angry Vegan *[aNGgrē vēgən]*: As ironic as it may sound, angry vegans are everywhere. Hell-bent on not only attacking meat eaters for their choices, but also attacking other vegans for their choices. The Angry Vegan will boast about their veganism and tear down anyone who holds a lower ranking in veganism. The Angry Vegan has such a prominent presence in vegan society, I've dedicated an entire chapter to them in this book. Mostly to help calm them down.

Beegan Vegan *[bēgən vēgən]*: There is a new breed of vegan out there who is so lazy (see Lazy Vegan, below) that they can't bring themselves to eliminate honey from their diets. These new Beegan Vegans conveniently look the other way in regard to stealing honey from bees so they can drop a bit o' honey in their tea or, perhaps, buy bread that has honey as an added ingredient. As far as I'm concerned, a Beegan Vegan is hardly a vegan.

Cheatin' Vegan *[CHētin' vēgən]*: The name says it all. These vegans cheat. Still call themselves vegan but know in their hearts they truly aren't. They may think they are *trying*, but they're really not even close. If you can consciously consume an animal, you're *not* vegan. They've been known to marry cauliflower but have steak on the side. You can always spot a Cheatin' Vegan; they smell like bacon.

Dietary Vegan *[dīə‚terē vēgən]*: Unlike Ethical Vegans (see below), the Dietary Vegan has learned the benefits of a whole-foods, plant-based diet (see below) and are vegan for their health, as opposed to for the animals. I started out as a Dietary Vegan. Over time, many of these vegans will make "the connection" and realize that wearing leather or supporting animal testing isn't a requirement of anyone's happy life, and they'll likely transition onto the next phase.

Ethical Vegan *[eTHək(ə)l vēgən]*: These vegans are in it for life and in it for the lives of animals. Each and every day, they make decisions about what they eat and wear and are compassionate and ethical in these decisions. To me, this is what being vegan is all about, and once you've arrived here, there is no "going back."

Former Vegan *[fôrmər vēgən]*: Oh, the Former Vegan. The countless individuals who, inevitably, when they find out you're vegan, say something like, "I *used* to be vegan." They spent years as a vegan and woke up an omnivore for whatever reason and rationale they can invent. Usually it's cheese. Sometimes it's sausage link. Might even be sausage-wrapped cheese balls. Or they say they just felt weak.

Freegan Vegan *[frēgun vēgən]*: A person who rejects consumerism and seeks to help the environment by reducing waste, especially by retrieving and using discarded food and other goods. They are vegan until confronted with food that would otherwise be thrown away. They are not vegan at all unless that food being thrown away is vegan.

Gluten-Free Vegan *[glootn frē vēgən]*: People who have celiac disease or suffer from gluten intolerance *and* are vegan, are Gluten-Free Vegans. It hardly seems possible to enjoy life as a gluten-free vegan, but guess what. It's just as easy as being vegan. There are so many gluten-free options available today that being a gluten-free vegan isn't a struggle, and you may actually feel better for adopting this diet. There is very little nutritional value in gluten (although seitan is such an amazing meat substitute that it would be foolish to not worship seitan).

High Carb Vegan *[hī kärb vēgən]*: Like the Starch Solution Vegan (see below), the High Carb Vegan loads up on carbs. These same vegans more than likely have a way to actually *burn* these carbs, so they are most likely athletic. Or overweight.

Instagram Vegan *[in-stuhgram vēgən]*: "Camera Eats First" is the motto of the Instagram Vegan. Shoot first, eat later. These vegans are proud to display their own culinary expertise or share an amazing meal they're eating at a restaurant to upload to the world, demonstrating that veganism *is* everywhere and delicious. There are hundreds of vegans to follow on Instagram, but I recommend you start with @VeganFatKid, and always use the hashtag #vegansofig.

Junk Food Vegan *[jəNGk food vēgən]*: Guilty. So, so guilty of this. Just as it sounds, the Junk Food Vegan finds and eats all the amazing things to eat that are either "accidentally vegan" or made as a delicious vegan version of something you already love. They replace many of the foods they used to love with not-always-so-healthy substitutes. Junk Food Vegans are known to eat a lot of meat replacers, macaroni and cheese, potato chips, and vegan ice cream. Also there's a flavor of Doritos (spicy sweet chili) that is accidentally vegan. And it tastes like Doritos.

Kombucha Vegan *[kôm ˈboōCHə vēgən]*: Six words—man buns and shoes with toes.

Lazy Vegan *[lāzē vēgən]*: Surest sign of a Lazy Vegan? They don't bother to read the labels or ask for a list of ingredients. They look the other way with honey or bone char sugar. They don't really care about the source of D3 or what "natural flavors" means on their soy vanilla creamer. "Meh, I'm Vegan," is their motto.

Militant Vegan *[mil-i-tuh nt vēgən]*: Militant vegans take Angry Vegans to the pavement. These are the ones who will ironically dress in camouflage and believe they are morally superior to people who eat meat, as well as other vegans. Their commitment to their lifestyle allows them to attack others verbally and sometimes even physically. They are a contradiction to true veganism.

Mostly Vegan *[mōs(t)lē vēgən]*: These may be at the bottom of the vegan food ladder. If anyone claims to be "mostly vegan" they most likely aren't even a little bit vegan. Actual vegans can't "look the other way" with their choices, and the mostly vegan individual wants to act like a vegan but knowingly deviates from the vegan agenda. The Mostly Vegan will politely eat meat at someone's house, never once mentioning being mostly vegan.

New Vegan *[n(y)oō vēgən]*: Yes! The pimply-faced vegan virgin. The thick-glasses-wearing newbie who can actually claim, "I've been vegan for a week." These are the next generation of vegan leaders and should be given an extra hug on National Hug a Vegan Day (September 23). Many New Vegans are pushed over the edge by watching documentaries on factory farming and "see the light." If you're reading this book and are thinking of becoming our newest member, call me and I'll personally hug you over the phone.

Oreo Vegan *[ôrē͵ō vēgən]*: Pop Tarts and Oreos are vegan (see page 201 for a more in-depth discussion on Oreos), as are countless other desserts and sweets. These Oreo Vegans are in love with chocolate and, once they find out they can eat it all, won't give it up. Take two frozen bananas, two cups of cold soy milk, four Oreos, and a tablespoon of peanut butter, and blend on high speed with a few ice cubes until it becomes a Peanut Butter Oreo Shake. The Oreo Vegan will post photos of the newest Oreo cookie flavor and usually use the caption: "Squeeeeeeee!"

Pumped Up Vegan *[pəmpt up vēgən]*: There are some massive vegan bodybuilders out there. In fact, Patrik Baboumian, the strongest man in all of Germany, is vegan. One of the United States' winningest UFC fighters, Nate Diaz, is vegan, and there are numerous football players, arm wrestlers, marathon runners, gymnasts, Olympians, and boxers who are vegan. These are the vegans we need on our side. They are living proof of everything you've read about: being vegan is the best diet for optimal health and, obviously, for the health of animals.

Quinoa Vegan *[keen-wah vēgən]*: Eat those superfoods! Quinoa and kale are the two most popular ingredients in a long list of superfoods. Goji berries and seaweed are also superfoods, but they don't taste great together in a smoothie. Technically, *superfoods* is a marketing term, but it does point aspiring health food nuts to amazing plant-based foods with incredible health-boosting properties.

Raw Vegan *[rô vēgən]*: A raw vegan eats a plant-based diet of uncooked (no hotter than 118°F) fruits and vegetables. This is also referred to as Level 10 Vegan, or veganism turned up to 11. I know a few raw vegans, and they prosper on this diet physically, but I always feel like they're probably not much fun at parties, if you know what I mean. As much as I know this is probably the healthiest human diet, I love my burgers, fries, and pizza too much to go raw.

Starch Solution Vegan *[stärCH sə ˈlooSH(ə)n vēgən]*: Eat those beautiful potatoes! The Starch Solution Vegan eats a plant-based diet that is high in starchy foods. It goes against any other diet notion, but it works. Plus, you get to eat potatoes.

Straight Edge Vegan *[streyt-ej vēgən]*: See, sXe or signified XXX or X. A subculture of hardcore punk, people who consider themselves straight edge refrain from using alcohol, tobacco, and other recreational drugs, often in reaction to the excesses of punk. For some, this extends to refraining from engaging in promiscuous sex, following a vegetarian diet, and/or not using caffeine or prescription drugs. Up the ante once more on straight edge by cutting out meat, dairy, and eggs, and you become a straight edge vegan.

Transitioning Vegan *[tran-zish-uhning vēgən]*: This might be you. Or this might be someone you know. A vegetarian taking that final step or an omnivore who is trying their hardest to go vegan. Of all the types of vegans, this is my favorite. Because they are trying. They are in a cocoon and are about to burst out a full-fledged vegan butterfly. (Technically, butterflies don't actually eat, they suck. Nectar. I don't think a 100 percent nectar diet is best for human health.)

Unsalted Vegan *[un sawl-tid vēgən]*: Like the Whole-Foods, Plant-Based Vegan (see below), the Unsalted Vegan avoids salt, as well as sugar, in their meals. There are so many incredible spices, including Mrs. Dash, that you can add to any dish to give it extra flavor, and salt can almost always be replaced. It's always best to cut back on the salt, unless it's on the rim of a glass.

VB6 Vegan *[vee bee six vēgən]*: A few years ago, a certain *New York Times* food writer and chef, who has since left the newspaper, wrote a controversial book called *VB6: Vegan Before Six*. The idea was that you could/should eat vegan, or plant-based, meals all day long, and then after 6:00 p.m., you could eat meat. While the concept *may* sound like an ideal approach, the idea that you can "shut off" being vegan is ridiculous, since it's a *lifestyle* and not a diet.

Whole-Foods, Plant-Based (WFPB) Vegan *[hōl foods plahnt beysd vēgən]*: If you've never read *The China Study* or watched *Forks Over Knives*, they are great places to begin to learn about the incredible health benefits of a WFPB diet. The most famous proponent of this diet remains Dr. T. Colin Campbell, who cowrote *The China Study* with his son Dr. Tom Campbell. This pioneering book reports on the findings of an important study of nutrition in China but also does much more. It summarizes laboratory studies and natural experiments from all over the world. The outcomes are unbelievable, except they're backed by science. It's fascinating and begins to prove that humans are natural herbivores. Antonym: Junk Food Vegan.

X-Vegan *[ecks vēgən]*: An X-Vegan is a former vegan who has been voted off the island. Excommunicated. These are usually well-known vegans who make a huge deal about all the reasons they started eating meat again. Unlike Former Vegans (above), X-Vegans will never come back. They've made up their minds. They are as sure about *not* being vegan as I am about *being* vegan. Vegans try their best to ignore this group and let them assimilate back into omnivorism and oblivion.

Yoga Vegan *[yoh-guh vēgən]*: Sometimes these are the toughest vegans to talk to because they spend 90 percent of their time on their head (or in some other outrageous pose). Yoga and veganism seem to travel together. And meditation. These promote a healthy and peaceful attitude, and I will probably never take part in either of them.

Zombie Vegan *[zämbē vēgən]*: Besides Rob Zombie, the filmmaker who happens to be vegan, there's also The Vegan Zombie, who operates a YouTube channel out of a secure bunker near Syracuse, New York. Rest assured, when the zombie apocalypse happens, that's where you'll find me. Not that I think Chris and Jon, the two men behind the brand, would be much protection (they are vegan, after all), but the boys can cook!

I am pretty sure I met one of each of these vegans that year at Vegetarian Summerfest, which is just one of hundreds of vegan conferences, events, and festivals that are popping up in every major city in the world. These events feature incredible food, samples, speakers, and giveaways and should be on any vegan's to-do list at least once a year. From the LA Vegan Beer and Food Festival to the NYC VegFest, these events are growing by leaps and bounds. How much are they growing? Well, the LA Vegan Beer Fest had such an incredible first year on the streets of LA that it had to move to a *much* bigger venue—the Rose Bowl Stadium in Pasadena. Now that's big.

And these numbers aren't only reflected in the United States. In May of 2016, it was reported that the number of vegans in the United Kingdom grew a whopping 360 percent over the past decade and Berlin has been rated the number one vegan-friendly city in Europe! People everywhere are recognizing the incredible health benefits, wide array of delicious foods, and the cruel ways in which animals are treated even in a "humane" setting.

Veganism is on the rise. Alvin Roth, Nobel Prize–winning economist and professor at Stanford and Harvard, predicts that veganism will become a dominant lifestyle in the very near future. His actual words are that "meat eating might become repugnant" to the general population.

I couldn't agree more.

A man can live and be healthy without killing animals for food; therefore, if he eats meat, he participates in taking animal life merely for the sake of his appetite.
—Leo Tolstoy

An entire book could be written on the vast array of questions new, or uninformed, vegans ask other vegans. I am going to attempt to compress the best of these questions into this one chapter. The following are actual questions that have been asked over the years by new, struggling, or simply uneducated vegans.

Are bananas vegan? Somewhere someone was told that bananas may be sprayed with a chemical derived from shrimp and crab shells. This, supposedly, allows bananas to stay fresh for a longer period of time. Unfortunately, this actually could be the case with some nonorganic bananas, so if you want to avoid it, buy organic. And before this practice stops, in the meantime you may want to avoid crab-shell-shellacked bananas. However, the banana itself *is* vegan.

Can I raise my dog vegan? Yes. Our SPCA rescue dog, Mandu, is vegan. The oldest dog in the world was vegan. Dogs are scavengers who hunt opportunistically. They also drink from the toilet opportunistically, but the less said about that the better. Anyway, dogs thrive on a vegan diet, just as humans do. It's good for them. Cats, on the other hand, are hunters/carnivores. Although some vegans report success with maintaining their cats on a vegan diet with supplements, the weight of informed opinion suggests that the felines probably require meat to stay healthy (and, more important, happy). Just try taking a mouse from a hungry cat. A note about domesticated pets: adopt, don't shop.

Is breast milk vegan? Yes. Breast milk (which is usually reserved for babies under three, by the way) *is* vegan. Same species, with consent. Same is true for semen and other bodily fluids. Vegan. *Same species, with consent.* If you consume either of these *without* consent, we may have to notify the authorities.

My neighbor has happy hens. Can I eat the eggs? If you want to, I can't stop you. But you're not vegan if you do. Even if a hen walked into your living room on its own volition, laid an egg, and then got in a car and drove itself to a farm sanctuary to live out its life—and you decided to eat that egg . . . you're not vegan. Now if that same chicken called you later on her chicken cell phone and was like, "I think I dropped an egg at your house, feel free to eat it," *then* you can eat it. Always remember, though, unless confronted with a cell phone–owning and talking chicken, vegans don't consume eggs (or meat or dairy). Of course, you might be thinking that eating the eggs of a happy hen next door is consistent with the *spirit* of veganism, but if so you'd be mistaken. Where did those hens come from? No, that's not the beginning of the age-old riddle about which came first, it's a real question. And the answer is invariably a *hatchery*. Now ask yourself what happened to the rooster chicks who were hatched in the hatchery. Lather. Rinse. Repeat.

Are Oreos vegan? Yes. So are almost all potato chips, Sour Patch Kids, and some PopTarts. There is so much vegan junk food out there that I bet you could trick an omnivore into becoming vegan just by feeding them junk food alone (can someone say "french fries"?). Keep in mind that you will not lose weight and your health will not improve if all you eat are Oreos and Sour Patch Kids. Everything in moderation.

Someone told me that plants feel pain. Is this true? No. Plants have no central nervous system or brain. Look at it this way: would you take your kids strawberry picking for the weekend or to the local slaughterhouse? There. Is. No. Comparison. Lettuce doesn't scream. Broccoli doesn't cower in the corner when you come at it with a knife. Corn *does* stalk, though.

Can kids be raised vegan? Yes, just don't feed them meat, eggs, dairy, or honey—and guess what. They're vegan. And they are going to thrive! It's the healthiest way to live. They will thank you one day for giving them this healthy head start, and they will truly be compassionate adults who love animals for life. We asked our three-year-old if he knew what being vegan meant, and he answered, "We don't eat animals." This makes it all worth it.

What about soy? Is it safe to eat? Yes: as mentioned earlier, you can safely consume up to five servings a day. Soy is loaded with protein, which is why the meat industry is trying its hardest to make everyone fear soy. It is a good source of various minerals such as calcium, iron, magnesium, phosphorus, potassium, sodium, zinc, copper, and manganese, and in its organic/non-GMO state, it's good for you and delicious. Soy is a bean. Beans are good for you.

Do I need to take supplements when I am vegan? B12 for sure. A vegan multivitamin might be helpful too, although doctors disagree about that. You may want to occasionally get checked for vitamins B12 and D (which you can get from standing in the sun for ten minutes a day). Other than these, you will be more than healthy enough eating whole grains, fruits, vegetables, and even the occasional vegan junk food. I said *occasional.*

Since becoming vegan six months ago, I seem to be tired all the time. What should I do? Sleep more.

I find myself having cravings for meat. What should I do? Stop kidding yourself. Your cravings for "meat" might be satisfied with meaty vegan alternatives. Listen, maybe you've been lured by the promise of a healthy diet by going vegan, and that's great, but there really is no such thing as a *vegan who craves meat*; more accurately, it's like saying you're a vegan who craves eating an animal. *It's not possible.*

Eat more veggies. Take your time. Replace items one by one. (Many experts will tell you to start by cutting out the dairy. By the way, milk is pretty much the worst thing on the planet for you, and it has been said that there is more rape, torture, and death in one glass of milk than there is in an entire steak.)

I'd like to add here that we *do* want as many new vegans as possible to come over. Give it a try. Ask as many questions as you need to if it helps maintain a cruelty-free lifestyle. Becoming vegan takes effort and commitment, and becoming an ethical vegan takes even more time. But it's worth it. For you. The planet. And, the animals.

If you wrote something for which someone sent you a check,
if you cashed the check and it didn't bounce, and if you then
paid the light bill with the money, I consider you talented.
—Stephen King

Part of my vegan experience was starting my own blog, MeatyVegan.
com. An online place to share my vegan experience, delectable recipes, interviews with other vegans, and scathing satire to entertain
and inform readers about my own life changes as I became vegan.
I've built a solid following and have made countless connections and
friends because of this blog. Companies shower me in their products
to review, and I've actually made some valued, professional, lifelong
connections because of it. The book you're reading is a direct result of
my blog.

You will find that the more time you spend as a vegan, the clearer
your own vegan voice will become. You will find where you fit in and,
perhaps, encourage others to go vegan, as well.

When I launched my blog, it was initially intended to document
my journey, not unlike this book. I wanted to explore how much of a
struggle veganism can be (when, in truth, it's the opposite), educate
and entertain others so they can make decisions about going vegan, or,
in many instances, provide diligent response to reader comments and
opinions that argued against veganism.

One of the first opponents to confront me was a man in Wales who
went by the nickname "The Angry Vegetarian."

The Angry Vegetarian wrote a guest blog post supporting his own
stance on veganism. He included hard-hitting thoughts such as: "If
you're a vegan, and you want to impose/impregnate your values onto
non-vegans, then please . . . please . . . please . . . please question the very
fabric and foundation of your lifestyle choice, because, trust me, there
will be flaws . . . many flaws. . . ." He continued, "And when you iron those
flaws out and become the perfect human being, you will have my full,
undivided, and unconditional attention."

His thinking was rational. How could anyone call themselves vegan
when they still get flu shots? Or drive a car? Or eat vegetables that

actually may have small bugs tucked between the leaves? Is it possible to really be 100 percent vegan?

Yes. It is. If you define veganism realistically. Veganism is about doing the *very best* you can do, on a daily basis. Thinking about your actions before taking action and taking into account the well-being of others, including animals. Or, perhaps, *especially* the animals.

A few months later, I learned that Michael, the Angry Vegetarian, went vegan. All in. I asked him if our interaction had some impact on this huge, life-changing decision, and he angrily said, "No."

The next day, he messaged me back and not-so-angrily said, "Yes."

Helping him think through his own dietary and lifestyle choices and learning from my own when making the decision to go vegan will remain one of the highlights of my personal journey, and one of the reasons I continued with my blog. A year later, I asked him what he felt is the best part about being vegan.

"Waking up every morning without having blood on my hands, and that I have finally found an honest affinity with animals," he said.

Michael and I are now good mates, and we keep in touch every day, still inspiring and supporting each other.

Of all my posts on my blog, the two that remain the most popular are the satirical piece I wrote about a ninety-four-year-old man "dying from veganism" and, surprisingly, one I wrote seeking "Conservative Republican Vegans." I noted that I had never met a vegan who is politically conservative. Veganism is not political, in fact it's more often compared to a religion, but the beliefs and general stereotypes of a conservative seem to go against most of the vegans I personally know. Take everything that veganism stands for, the high-octane version of the vegan lifestyle that covers everything from simple diet changes to Ahimsa. Could you subscribe to a diet without meat, dairy, and eggs and still be a conservative? Possibly. But the *entire* vegan lifestyle? No. The two ideals are polar opposites. I couldn't imagine a conservative Republican getting behind the charter of a jet transporting 750 hens from California to the Farm Sanctuary in Watkins Glen, New York. Or a conservative Republican wearing an "I Don't Eat Animals" T-shirt (unless they were trying to be sarcastic).

But, then again, the Republican party was founded by antislavery activists in 1854, and they established equal rights for all men (women would have to wait)—that seems pretty liberal. There is actually a website dedicated to moderate Republicans who are vegan. *The Vegan Republican* states on their homepage: "Everybody thinks vegans are always liberals. Not true. Some of us are moderate Republicans." They do feel compelled to mention that the online commentary needs to stay "mild."

The publisher of *Forbes*, Rich Karlgaard, is a Republican who wrote an excellent HuffPost article about being vegan. However, within the article he calls himself an "almost vegan." Of course, there is no such thing. So, *do* conservative vegans truly exist?

I didn't think so, but I was wrong. There are actually thousands of conservative vegans around the world, and the once-a-week response to this blog post is proof. Some of them are actually surprised I asked the question since, in their circles, the other vegans they know are conservative or vote Republican. One response that really seemed to sum it up for me was from this commenter:

> My family and I are 100 percent plant-based, conservative, Christian, Republicans. Yes, we are out here! We are all plant-based for health, and I am plant-based because I do not believe it is appropriate to kill and eat animals when we can healthfully live on plant foods. As a Christian, I believe biblically that God's perfect world is a plant-based one. Man and animal lived in harmony prior to 'the fall of man,' as can be read about in Genesis, where everyone was an herbivore during this time. It was only after 'the flood' of the earth that God 'allowed' meat eating. While he allowed it, he did not demand it nor did he state that is best for man to eat meat. Finally, upon Christ's return, 'the lion will lay with the lamb' once again; meaning everyone will once again be an herbivore; therefore, I believe biblically that God's perfect, harmonious world is one where all man and animal alike are herbivores/ vegan/plant-based.

As for the Republican side of me, I believe fully in the strength of the free market, and everyone without serious mental or physical disability being accountable for making their own way. No able-bodied individual should be allowed to ride freely on the hard work of others. However, on that note, we also believe in supporting financially, and are physically involved in, nearly ten charitable organizations, and we provide others jobs through our small business. Those who work to become 'the haves' or 'the wealthy' in this country are those who can support jobs, give to the needy, and generally provide others a better way of life than the government ever can. The free market supports success for all, while a socialist society supports everyone being at a disadvantage. In a socialist-based society, no one has the incentive to work hard because it will all be taken away, and when that happens, it also leaves nothing for those seeking a handout. Everyone is poor and downtrodden in this scenario.

This response proved to me that veganism is compatible through any range of religious and political beliefs. Being vegan is a choice you make in the interest of either your health or animal welfare (perhaps some make the choice for the environment, which is also admirable). You can vote for whomever you like and still care enough about animals to want to protect and not eat them. You can believe in Second Amendment Rights and never own or fire a gun at another living being, all the while still supporting animal sanctuaries. You can be pro-life and be, well, pro-life.

You *can* believe in God and be vegan.

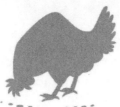

17

HOW TO GO VEGAN
IN TWO EASY STEPS

*You have just dined, and however scrupulously the slaughterhouse
is concealed in the graceful distance of miles, there is complicity.*
—*Ralph Waldo Emerson*

Step one: Stop eating meat, dairy, and eggs.
Step two: Stop wearing wool, leather, and silk.

It's that easy! You're now vegan! Congratulations!

Well, at least in theory it's that easy. Some people have a harder time giving things up. Tastes, traditions, habits, family, and friends all come into play when you're making a radical life change such as going vegan. Allow yourself time.

It is worth it.

When I finally quit smoking after almost twenty years, it was immediate. I was traveling back from London with a friend who smoked a pack a day, and I witnessed him going into shock over not being able to smoke during the eight-hour flight. His hands were sweating. His heart was racing. He was going through withdrawal. Once we landed at Heathrow, we made our way to the terminal. He had to lie on the airport floor for nearly twenty minutes to regroup. I stood over him as three airport security guards insisted we call an ambulance. All the while, he panted, "I'm fine. I'm fine." As soon as he was up and out the door, he lit a cigarette. While I did smoke some Chesterfields in the pubs while playing pool "English style," as soon as we arrived back in New York a week later, I knew I had smoked my last cigarette. I would never smoke again. I was scared straight and quit cold turkey. Or, as we vegans like to say, cold "Tofurky." (By the way, Tofurky makes an incredible line of delicious vegan products, and I've partied with the company owners in California. The food at the event was not what I was expecting; they ordered vegan pizza.)

When you tell someone you've quit smoking, they immediately congratulate you. When you tell someone you've quit eating meat, dairy, eggs, and honey, they inevitably ask, "Where do you get your protein?"

Years later, I essentially did the same with alcohol, quitting drinking as I did smoking. I remember being out on the town with nondrinkers and seeing them having as much fun as I was without getting drunk, and certainly without the next day's hangover. I didn't need that in my life, so on my forty-third birthday, I quit. I decided that I had consumed enough alcohol to last me a lifetime and that I'd rather be healthier during the second half of my life. I realized I didn't *need* alcohol in my system. It was making me see double and think single.

When you tell someone you've quit drinking, they always ask why, or assume you had a problem and congratulate you. When you tell someone you've quit eating milk, dairy, and eggs, they assume that it's a phase and that you'll soon return to eating meat, since it's such an important part of a healthy diet.

These decisions are for the betterment of your health; you can make the switch at any point in your life. It's never too late, until it's too late. If you could add quality years to your life, would you? If these years included living a more compassionate life, wouldn't you want that, too? Change can happen.

When making these radical changes and especially when transitioning to veganism, allow yourself to make mistakes, even if they are by mistake. Take your time. Read labels. Ask others for advice, and embrace the new you.

Go on. Embrace you. No one's looking.

Learn from my experience: it's all going to seem overwhelming at first, and you may not feel the positive health benefits right away. In fact, I was vegan for five months when a letter I wrote to *VegNews* magazine was published. In it, I essentially griped about how I had been promised a world of positive changes, and none of these miraculous things were taking place:

Dear Laura Hooper Beck,
I went 100-percent vegan from a 100-percent omnivore lifestyle. I had just planned to try out the thirty-day Vegan Challenge, but it's become a longer commitment. It's exciting, but I have to say that I feel exactly the same as I did before making the switch. Is there a way for you to assure me that continuing on the vegan path will result in all the health benefits I was promised?
—*Incredulous in Ithaca*

The reply:

First off, congrats on going vegan. You're the greatest. I think there are two things at play here. The first could be that you're getting healthy internally, even if you haven't lost a billion pounds or picked up the ability to fly. The second is that you might just feel pretty much the same. Maybe you'll get sick less often in the future (I haven't had a cold in years, which, honestly, is better than being able to fly), or maybe you won't. Sure, eating vegan is better for you than the Standard American Diet of chemical-laden cheese-like products and meat laced with feces and pesticides, but it's not a cure all. Here's what I think—being vegan is about not supporting the industries that put profit above everything else, while still eating delicious food. I'm not a religious or spiritual person, but I do believe then when you eat dead animals, you are ingesting all of the fear and suffering they went through in their lives, and that shiz cannot be good for you. Besides, I really don't want to be haunted by a turkey; those fools are crazy.

This letter ran in the October 2012 issue. I had been vegan for just over a year and was still seeking all the fringe benefits of the lifestyle. My body was still going through a change.

And then it started to happened. A month or so later, I started losing weight. Not a billion pounds exactly, but I could feel myself becoming lighter, and my pants weren't getting any tighter. Over time, on a vegan diet, I lost a total of thirty pounds of extra weight I obviously didn't need. Four notches on my belt. Being vegan did have a positive impact on my overall health.

In fact, there was one extra *big* bonus I didn't see coming.

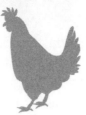

18

EATING PLANTS IS SEXY: MAKING VEGAN BABIES

We have reason to believe that man first walked
upright to free his hands for masturbation.
—Lily Tomlin

Cue the porn music. Bow chicka wow wow.

A little-known fringe benefit about being vegan that's really rather hard to ignore: *your sex life is going to improve.* Dramatically. There's a long list of reasons sex is better as a vegan, from weight loss and more energy to your skin and hair improving and even body fluids tasting better. There is actually a fun, and tasty, pineapple experiment you can try for your next date night (Google it).

Especially when all you eat are delicious plants, there is no question as to why rabbits reproduce at the rate they reproduce—you just have to. Lettuce mate. In fact, feeding yourself juicy, erotic, colorful fruits and firm, crunchy, crispy vegetables will have such a positive impact on your body that it might just get you, and your partner, aroused.

Salads are sexy. Nothing beets a good time.

The medical condition known as erectile dysfunction (ED), which occurs when a man has consistent and repeated problems sustaining an erection, is most often caused by clogged arteries. Up to 50 percent of men in their fifties suffer from ED. Arteries that, for years, have been coated with plaque (cholesterol) from meat, eggs, and dairy. These arteries, which are engineered to pump blood quickly through your body, now resemble a clogged sewer. Blood is trying its hardest to flow, and this is where your penis comes in. If you're a guy.

If you're a straight cis woman, this would be where someone else's penis comes in. And, if you're a lesbian cis woman, I apologize for all of the penis talk. Anyway, where was I?

Oh, yes. Your penis. Your penis works best when it has a fast, uninterrupted flow of blood circulating into it. Slower blood, limper results. In fact, many men who are prescribed Viagra® for ED are also prime candidates for massive heart attacks.

If blood isn't flowing down there, it isn't flowing everywhere else. Men can actually have a healthy libido, an urge and desire to have sex, and not get a response from "down under." All the foreplay in the world won't clear clogged arteries.

Meat eaters experience a much higher rate of heart disease/clogged arteries, whereas vegans, as you can probably guess, have little issue in this department. In fact, ever since man first walked erect, fruits and vegetables have been the best natural artery-clearing remedy.

Fruits and vegetables rarely come with a warning label. Few doctors prescribe sick patients "more red meat."

There is, however, a *six-page* warning label for Viagra®. Personally, I'd rather have a salad and a night of sex than a heart attack.

While switching entirely to a vegan diet might seem radical for a lot of omnivores (and, as we all know, vegetarians cannot give up cheese . . . they're such wieners), I'd personally consider it less drastic than taking a blue pill to get an erection that also causes 16 percent of users to get a headache. So, there you are with a ten-dollar erection, and you still have to say, "Not tonight dear, I have a headache."

Not a fan of taking drugs for sex? Well, then, you can always pump it up. Simply place your penis inside a specially-designed cylinder— and begin pumping. The pump draws air out of the cylinder, creating a vacuum around the penis, causing it to fill with blood, leading to an erection. An elastic band worn around the base of the penis maintains the erection during intercourse.

This is an actual thing. A penis pump. And while it might lead to a good time, as a tool to get it up, it's not what most people would consider foreplay.

You can try these methods—or you could just go vegan and eat a beauteous bounty of fruits and vegetables and, when the time is right, be ready to go.

Consuming fruits and vegetable *also* increases serotonin levels— the happiness chemical—which can quickly lead to the desire to have more sex. According to a 2012 *Nutrition Journal* study, people who don't consume *any* meat tend to be happier overall and less stressed than those who do. Researchers attributed this phenomenon to the presence of fatty acids, specifically arachidonic acid—animal source of Omega-6 fatty acids—which can cause mood-disturbing changes in the brain at high levels.

Eating fruits and vegetables = sexy. Eating the body parts of dead animals = not sexy.

Also, keep in mind, plants and plant-derived foods contain *no cholesterol*. Within a few months to a year, you'll start to feel these amazing health benefits every day, and you can take this newfound energy and enthusiasm to bed with you.

I did, and now I have a baby to prove it.

Since I had a low sperm count following a vasectomy reversal, Jen and I were trying to conceive for a few years. I am not sure I could have ever sustained daily sex (you read it right) without plants powering my passion and performance. During this whole time, we were fostering our infant son, and as soon as we knew he was freed for adoption, boom. I knocked her up. Jen had just turned forty, and we both attribute our sex drive, having sex every day (Every. Day.) and the ability to conceive "later in life" to our vegan diets. I became a forty-something dad of two-under-two.

Looking to make a baby? Are you nuts? According to Dr. Greger, a diet high in walnuts will also increase the quantity and quality of sperm. And, as mentioned earlier, the higher the saturated fat intake, such as meat, the lower the sperm count. And for women, being vegan results in increased natural lubrication.

Get where I'm going here?

If you love sex, you'll love being vegan. If you love steaks more than sex, you may want to talk to someone. Suffice to say, if you want to continue eating meat and are content with your mundane sex life, that's on you. But know that a diet rich in fruits and vegetables and antioxidants will make those million little swimmers healthier, and it will give them the straightest, fastest luge to shoot through.

And who doesn't love the luge?

> *It's never really been that hard for me. I've never had any desire to eat meat. In fact, when I was a kid I would have a really difficult time eating meat at all.*
> —*Tobey Maguire*

If you think being vegan is a challenge as an adult, imagine being a baby.

When Jen and I decided to have a family, we tried to conceive for a few years. As a backup plan, we became foster parents with the hope of one day adopting. Our first placement was twin boys. We went from zero babies to two seven-month-olds and had to buy or borrow two of everything.

While these boys were in our care for four months, we were feeding them a vegan diet until they could be reunited with their older brother. During that time, their pediatrician remarked on their significant progress and development. They were hearty, healthy, happy boys, and we were happy to feed them a whole-foods, plant-based diet.

Then, in March 2013, we got a call to foster a newborn baby boy. We picked him up from the hospital when he was five days old. We took Luke home and were instant parents of a beautiful baby boy. A baby boy we began raising vegan. As the months passed and the details of his adoption were being solidified, Jen became pregnant. Damn vegan stamina. We can't say that Leia was "an accident" because we had been trying for years, but as soon as we stopped "officially" trying, she came into being. The conception happened on the night of Jen's fortieth birthday party. Happy birthday!

In nine months, Jen gave birth and Luke became a big brother, and the number of vegan babies in the house had suddenly doubled.

The interesting part of our stay at the hospital was the meals. When a new baby is born, the hospital treats the parents to a steak dinner. There you are, in a hospital, being given what may very well be the number one reason most people are there in the first place.

Of course, since we were vegans and Jen was also gluten-free, the celebratory meal wasn't quite as elaborate. I ordered takeout Thai food.

Every day, you are provided a card to fill out, indicating either your preferred selections or your dietary restrictions. So, each day we would indicate gluten-free and vegan, and each day we were overwhelmed with what we received—sarcasm.

Lifting the cloche on day one revealed a baked potato. Now, I love potatoes, but even I was a little disappointed with this potato. It looked sad. Almost as sad as day two's "meal."

A bowl of rice.

Day three was another potato. (Thankfully, a different potato.)

This pattern continued for most of our stay, since the system in the kitchen was entirely based on mathematics. A computer would eliminate all food that wasn't vegan and further eliminate all food that wasn't gluten-free, and finally it would spit out a card for the dietary worker to put the results of this equation on a plate.

I would run down to the cafeteria to see what might be gluten-free and vegan and would come back with, you guessed it, potato chips or french fries. Hospitals have a long way to go toward accommodating patients' needs, and, needless to say, we ended up getting takeout or delivery the entire time we were there.

Once home, though, we were a new vegan family of four settling in for the winter.

Of course, at that point Leia was being breastfed (where Luke couldn't be), and to help bring up her weight, we were supplementing her diet with organic soy formula. Breast milk is best for newborn babies, and there is no 100 percent vegan baby formula on the market (it contains vitamin D3, which is not vegan); however, we had to feed both Luke and Leia the highest-quality organic soy formula we could find during the early days of their development.

When our baby was born, I made the announcement on social media and fielded the usual questions about raising newborn vegan babies and dealt with comments about whether breast milk is vegan. I usually ignore these comments, but one comment I couldn't ignore was about raising vegan babies in the first place. After all, we had previously fostered the twins and fed them a vegan diet while they were with us (which, by the way, is its own controversy) and now had every intention of raising our son and new baby vegan.

"Shouldn't your kids be given 'the choice' of whether or not to be vegan?" a friend asked, obviously trying to stir things up a bit.

Of course, there are a few things wrong with what this person was saying:

1. Breastfeeding babies are vegan already, and when they transition to other milk, plant-based milk is better for them than dairy milk.
2. When babies transition to solid foods, the best diet for them is plant-based, and nearly all baby food is made from fruits and vegetables anyway. Starting a one-year-old on bacon (even bacon that has been pulverized in a blender) is not recommended by most doctors.
3. Babies don't have jobs or make money or go grocery shopping, so they will eat whatever they are given and what's available to them; plus, why shouldn't this be the healthiest diet possible?
4. As parents, we all naturally make "a choice" for our babies (who can't speak or choose) when we feed them food (vegan or not). Bottom line? Children don't have (and shouldn't have) choices at a young age. Parents know what's best. Once they become defiant teens, then that's a different story.

Giving them a choice to select their diet would be the same as giving them the choice to wear sunscreen or not. Are you going to wait until they can make their own decisions on whether or not to burn themselves to a crisp? No, of course not, you're protecting them from long-term health issues, and that's exactly what a vegan diet does for growing children.

This reminds me of the great Vegan Sidekick, a popular online vegan comic strip. The two-panel strip features a parent holding her little one's hand as she talks to another parent.

First panel:
Person one says, "I don't make my child eat meat."
Person two says, "Forcing your way of life on your children is extreme."

Second panel:
Person one says, "I make my child eat meat."
Person two says, "Forcing your way of life on your children is awesome."

It gets challenging, too, when we keep our two vegan-raised babies in a daycare. Their daycare is a nationally recognized and certified operation that has always received high marks for curriculum and care from six-week-old babies to pre-K kids, so having two in daycare isn't cheap. At one point, we were spending as much as two mortgages per month when it dawned on us that some of our hard-earned money was paying for the center's nonvegan snacks and dairy milk, while we were obligated to provide our own vegan snacks and soy milk for our kids. We decided to meet with the director to make change happen.

While it took almost a year of back-and-forth to convince them it was just as easy to buy a gallon of soy milk as it was to buy a gallon of dairy milk, we finally broke through, and now our kids (as well as other kids with dietary restrictions) have equity in snacking. (We never mentioned that our kids poo more, so they are actually more work.)

The daycare has also started a vegetable garden. Abundant with regional bounty, this quarter-acre patch of land teaches young children about where their food actually comes from. It dawned on me one day when I was picking the kids up that the daycare hadn't started a slaughterhouse.

Raising children on a plant-based diet gives them a head start on great health, and teaching them about veganism gives them a compassionate and loving outlook on all animals. Today we have two little vegans thriving on their plant-based diets. While Luke's friends are picky eaters who do not eat their veggies, it's literally all Luke eats. Nothing warms our heart more than to hear our four-year-old say, "We don't eat animals." And he says this with confidence.

As vegan parents, we are also always prepared to replace unvegan passages with vegan phrases in children's books and songs to reinforce the philosophy and lifestyle we want to instill in them from an early age.

"This Little Piggy went to market . . . this Little Piggy stayed home . . . this Little Piggy had kale salad." Or, "Baa baa, black sheep, have you any wool? No sir. No sir. It's not for you." That kind of thing.

After our second baby was born, friends of ours gave us a copy of Lois Ehlert's wonderful board book, *Eating the Alphabet*. Lois Ehlert's Caldecott-winning children's books are alive with vibrant colors. Her collages are just beautiful, and kids love them. So many of her books are a natural part of every infant's library and traditionally share a shelf with Eric Carle's *The Very Hungry Caterpillar*. The big, noticeable difference between Carle's gastronomic tome and Lois's *Eating the Alphabet* is that one book is vegan and the other . . . well, sorry caterpillar fans, is not.

The interesting thing about reading *Eating the Alphabet* out loud is that, unlike so many other books, it doesn't have to be edited on the fly. Lois Ehlert takes the reader from A to Z without once stopping at "C' is for chicken, or "P" is for pork, or "W" for water buffalo. To be even more specific, the author didn't use cheese or eggs. Everything in the book is edible for our little vegans.

To some, this might be overlooked, but to me the book conveys a very powerful message that resonates with me every time I read it: *Animals are not food.*

They just shouldn't be. There is no valid reason or argument to eat animals, and anyone who continues to do so is clearly not willing to make the connection. Animals are our friends, and we don't eat our friends. At least I don't, and our babies don't, either.

The gold standard for vegan children's books would have to be anything written and illustrated by Ruby Roth. I was first introduced to Ruby Roth's *Vegan Is Love: Having Heart and Taking Action* at a Friday Dinner. I was immediately drawn in by the amazing illustrations and further impressed with the excellent, bold writing. A children's book about being vegan? This was just what I needed (since most of the literature I personally read needs to have pictures).

Jen bought me *Vegan is Love* and *That's Why We Don't Eat Animals* for Christmas one year so I could read them over and over again to our kids. Sometimes I need help with the big words, but that's okay because the drawings are *so* good and I can point to the pictures. Ruby's books were the best I've read since *Steven the Vegan*, which is another must-have if you have kids. Ruby's one-of-a-kind illustrations are vibrant and colorful, her words are so meaningful, and most important, her books cover the important topics and issues about being kind to all animals and not hurting or eating them.

Not surprisingly, when *Vegan Is Love: Having Heart and Taking Action* came out, there were many people who were opposed to it. They didn't like being reminded about how poorly animals are treated and felt that the books could actually make kids pickier eaters by not wanting to eat animals. Imagine that? Teaching children to love all animals and letting them know there are options for food that don't include animals?

Ruby also wrote and illustrated *V Is for Vegan: The ABCs of Being Kind* and a hands-on cookbook for the little ones, *The Help Yourself Cookbook for Kids*. Excellent reading for your little vegan.

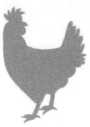

19

SPECIESISM AND THE HUMANE TOUCH

He who is cruel to animals becomes hard also in his dealings with men.
We can judge the heart of a man by his treatment of animals.
—Immanuel Kant

One of the more interesting dynamics of being vegan is being singled out. While I personally am lucky enough to have a safety net of numerous vegan friends, I still come up against omnivores on an almost daily basis and sometimes have to "defend my diet." Whether they need nutritional validation or they want to educate me on the virtues of dining on animals or perhaps it's how leather and wool are the warmest material for winter coats (which they aren't), omnivores have every known excuse in the book for consuming animals.

"So you're vegan now? You don't eat meat?" Jules said while we waited outside for a table at a local Thai Restaurant. Thai food, and many different kinds of Asian foods, are almost always available vegan. Rice. Noodles. Veggies. Some dumplings. Just watch out for fish sauce. At this particular restaurant, Jen orders the pho and I get a spicy crispy tofu served over rice that would rival any meat dish on any menu.

"No meat. Or dairy, eggs, or honey," I replied as I peered into the restaurant window to see if they were clearing a table or calling my name.

"I could never do that. I love meat too much, and I need the extra protein." This sort of reply is always accompanied by a somewhat apologetic, sheepish look. Inevitably, the conversation usually proceeds as follows:

"But I only eat grass-fed, hormone-free, humanely slaughtered animals," Jules went on. "I care enough about animals and my health to make sure what I'm eating is good for me and as good as possible for the animals."

As good as possible for the animals? What part of any of that is ever good for the animals?

The commonly agreed-upon definition of humane killing: "an animal must be either killed instantly or rendered insensible to pain until death supervenes." When killing animals for food, meaning slaughtering, this implies they must be stunned prior to bleeding out so they immediately become unconscious. None of the above sounds humane, and very little of this is practiced on a global scale.

"And I only eat a little red meat," she continued. (They always continue. At this point, we were both hoping this conversation wouldn't carry over to dinner.) A *little* red meat. A little portion of an entire cow. Do people realize that regardless of your own portion size, it still requires an entire dead animal? You could eat a single bite of sirloin or an entire twenty-four-ounce rib eye, and it still involved *one* entire cow being killed against its will, years before its natural life expectancy.

"There's actually no such thing as 'humanely slaughtered,'" I ended up saying. "That's a yuppie phrase to make you feel better about yourself."

"They can be. Raised happy and humanely slaughtered."

"I suppose they can be raised happy but isn't that the ultimate betrayal? Killing them after caring for them? Befriending and then beheading them?"

Long, awkward silence.

Finally, she said, "It's *my* choice to eat meat. I don't judge you about your diet."

These conversations always remind me of the time my mom, who is not vegan, mentioned that since she makes vegan foods available for us when we come over for dinner to her house, we should make meat available to *her* when she comes over to *our* house. As if we could suddenly look the other way cooking and serving a dead animal in our home?

Needless to say, my mom never comes over to our house.

Humanely slaughtered is an oxymoron. Like *jumbo shrimp* or *found missing.* Two words that, when placed together, negate each other. It makes no sense. Nonsense.

It's becoming evident that veganism is on the rise, and the meat and dairy industries are starting to feel the pinch. These powerful drivers of our economy are pandering to their audience and helping sway back in their direction anyone who may consider a vegan, or even vegetarian, diet. If you can feel good about the "sustainably sourced" salmon you are eating, you will feel like you are doing your part to help the planet, promote your health, and make strides toward eating animals in a more humane manner. All the while ignoring the truth that *animals are not food.*

I once posted an article about the sewage pools that exist outside of factory farms in North Carolina. These pools are filled to their shores with waste from the thousands of pigs being raised for food. At night, an orchestrated sprinkler system sprays the liquid into the air and surrounding neighborhoods near the farms. This toxic formula is causing countless health problems for people living in these areas, and even when these facts are clearly shown, someone inevitably says they only consume "sustainably raised, humanely slaughtered, grass-fed, free-range, happy, local pigs." Pigs that form bonds with the owners of the farm to eventually face the ultimate showdown that they cannot win.

While these smaller farms may seem more sustainable, they do as much damage to the planet as the larger farms do since there are more animals per acre. Not to mention these same people who claim to "only eat from their local farm" are also supporting the factory farms indirectly, unknowingly, and frequently when they order pizza covered in bacon and sausage from a national franchise.

They drink milk that comes from a dairy farm that drives the meat industry by killing male offspring for veal. They dine at popular restaurants that serve up to fifty million chicken wings per week. They spend their money on meat, dairy, and eggs every day without once stopping to consider that they are, in fact, supporting factory farms.

Being vegan means you're not. Ever.

A person I met through a professional network posted an online photo album of his kids visiting a nearby pig farm. It was one of those "pasture-raised" farms where pigs can lounge about happily and interact with visitors. The photos showed his daughter snuggling with some piglets and a family of pigs relaxing in the early summer sun. Rubbing one another's bellies. Eating vegan bonbons. Oinking. You know, doing pig things that pigs do in the wild.

The caption that accompanied the photos read something like: "Took the kids to the The Piggery to 'show them where their food comes from.'"

Where their food comes from? Pigs shouldn't be considered food. They are *animals*. Sentient beings like your dog or cat. Wait, am I missing something here? Is there more to this story?

I visited The Piggery's website and found this explanation of their pig "paradise" located on a seventy-acre farm in Trumansburg, just outside of Ithaca:

> Here at The Piggery, we're a different kind of farm. We're doing everything we can to create pork that is good for the people, good for the land, and good for the pigs, with a focus on minimizing our carbon footprint. We raise heirloom breeds of pigs on pasture, supplemented with locally raised GMO-free small grains (barley, wheat, triticale, peas).

Now I know I am missing something here. You can actually bring your kids to the farm to play with the piglets, who will, within a few months, be slaughtered for their meat. What part of this is "good for the pigs"?

"I'd like to eat this one, daddy," said the freckle-faced, pigtailed girl in the yellow summer sundress as she rubbed the belly of a six-month-old piglet. The pig let out a happy grunt as it scratched its back on the pebbles and dirt.

"How much for the piglet? The girl needs this one." The doting father turns to the farmer, checkbook and pen in hand. "Name your price."

"That little cutie is just a hundred dollars. But cut up properly, it is worth well over three hundred dollars. You'll get pork chops, ham hocks, center loin, spare ribs, and, of course, bacon."

"Brilliant! We'll take it! Honey, hand the little critter over to the nice man to have its head cut off."

"Thank you, daddy! I love you."

The site goes on to mention that they breed "handsome Mulefoot & Gloucestershire Old Spot boars with Yorkshire, Durcoc, Hampshire, and Tamworth ladies to make some darn cute piglets."

Are these people for real? What's the point of how cute they are if they are going to be slaughtered? Does the pig's level of cuteness somehow get them out of their death sentence? Imagine the farmer going, "Not cute. Slaughter. Not cute. Slaughter. Not cute. Slaughter. Cute. Let it live." Someone chooses life or death for these animals based on their snuggle-bility?

But, rest assured, you cute little pigs have nothing to fear—you're all being "humanely slaughtered." According to the site: "We have witnessed the slaughtering procedure and are comfortable that the slaughterhouse does a good, humane job." Happy (darn cute) pigs meeting the ultimate, untimely, unnecessary, unhappy end.

They should change their tagline to "We Put *Laughter* Back into Slaughter."

In the slaughtering of animals for food, there is no such things as a "humane killing." But, as it turns out, I happen to have firsthand, personal information on what an actual humane killing of an animal looks like when this path is chosen for a pet.

Jen always said that she didn't find her cat, Dubu; Dubu found *her*. A gorgeous long-haired, black-and-white tuxedo cat, Dubu traveled with her from her life in California to our lives in New York.

Dubu was Jen's very grounding force. Her comfort and her love. In many ways, I am convinced she loved Dubu more than me, and I honestly can't say I blame her. At twelve years of age, Dubu was diagnosed with inoperable and terminal injection-site sarcoma, and she was fading fast. The vet recommended that putting Dubu down was the best for her and offered to take care of it for us at Cornell. While the procedure at a world-class vet school is likely as humane as anywhere, Jen loved Dubu so much she decided to have her last moments with us. We opted for in-home euthanasia.

Whole Animal Veterinary Geriatrics and Hospice Services provides in-home euthanasia services for new clients, and Dr. Goldberg has a licensed social worker affiliated with the practice who provides counseling before, during, and after the procedure. It's as much support as you could ever need for going through the unthinkable. Jen met with the doctor, and they decided on a date.

It was very solemn and quiet in the apartment as three separate injections were given to Dubu while she slowly started to fall asleep for the last time. All the while, Jen fought back tears and I tried to be supportive. She held Dubu, comforted her, stroked her, and said her good-byes as the thirty-minute procedure came to an end, just like Dubu's amazing life.

This is as humane as it comes, and there is no cow, pig, chicken, turkey, or any other animal "humanely killed" for food that would ever be treated this way. None.

> *We need, in a special way, to work twice as hard to help people*
> *understand that the animals are fellow creatures,*
> *that we must protect them and love them as we love ourselves.*
> *—César Chávez*

The idea of *speciesism* is relatively new. From Dictionary.com:

speciesism (ˈspē-shēz-i-zəm)
1: prejudice or discrimination based on species; especially, discrimination against animals
2: the assumption of human superiority on which speciesism is based

The phrase originated in 1970 and was introduced by British psychologist Richard Ryder. Ryder argued that "since Darwin, scientists have agreed that there is no 'magical' essential difference between humans and other animals, biologically-speaking. Why then do we make an almost total distinction morally? If all organisms are on one physical continuum, then we should also be on the same moral continuum."

Darwin was no vegan, but his observations on the animal kingdom are legendary and help us, today, make these important distinctions regarding our shared planet. *Animals are not food (at least not to humans).* They are no more food than humans in this context. They have every right to live; and keeping, torturing, killing, skinning, and eating them is morally wrong. Animals deserve to live, have emotions, and feel pain, just like humans do.

Reread that last sentence.

There really should be no difference between humans and the rest of the animal kingdom, and the film *Speciesism* brings to light so many of these disconnects and provides the opportunity to take note of what nonvegans do, and support, on a daily basis to perpetuate this idea.

At what point in the animal kingdom do most people disconnect? Where does the line get drawn? They clearly have no issue eating pigs, cows, or chickens but won't eat dogs, horses, or parakeets (generally speaking). And what about pigs that are kept as pets?

It's like what Jon Stewart said on *The Daily Show* when Gene Baur, president of the Farm Sanctuary and author of *Living the Farm Sanctuary Life,* was a guest: "It's harder to eat meat when you know the animal's name." Jon and his wife now own a Farm Sanctuary in New Jersey.

Being vegan erases the line completely. *All* animals deserve to live.

I tell my vegan friends this and press on, "So then, *now* tell me why can't everyone be vegan?"

"Because a lot of people enjoy meat," they reply.

"A lot of animals enjoy life," I say. I'm done here.

The other day I was at our kids' daycare. I sat down at a tiny table in the "pretend" kitchen. In the center of the table was a fake, plastic roasted chicken. Seemed an odd choice for kids to play with, but I have to remember that others don't see the world through the same lens as I do. A friend's three-year-old daughter sat next to me.

She was pouring me pretend tea, being all sweet and innocent.

"Do you know what this is?" I asked her, pointing at the plastic chicken, knowing I was finally communicating to someone at the same intellectual level as myself. "It's a *dead* bird," I went on, not once thinking about how I could potentially scar her for life.

Without missing a beat, she replied, "No. It's a chicken."

Indoctrination starts early.

> *"Animals are my friends . . . and I don't eat my friends."*
> —*George Bernard Shaw*

The other day I was talking to a friend about the Kentucky Derby—the annual event where the one percent stand around in big hats drinking mint juleps and cheering on animals being abused by little people—and how horrible the sport and the conditions are for the horses. He countered my argument by insisting that it was an industry not unlike any other industry, and if people want to support the races, that's their right, their choice. He then continued talking about other industries, and the more he talked, the more I slowly started to wonder if he was kidding.

"I mean, horses are one thing. The same is true for pigs, chickens, or cows. Plus, do you ever stop to think about all of those farmers out of work and the farm supply companies? And the truckers and butchers? So to you, I would assume, it's better just to let them all die out than to strive for as humane treatment as possible?" he asked.

"What about butchers?" I answered his question with a question, something I could do all day.

"They would all go out of business. Are you opposed to small business, too?"

"Do you think I am?" See what I mean?

I watched and waited to see if he was kidding. He wasn't. He truly believed that raising animals to be slaughtered was perfectly fine and that we should *support* these activities in order to keep these businesses profitable. He continued.

"I have a friend who is dying from lung cancer, and still I don't think the tobacco industry should be boycotted. Other people's livelihoods, jobs, need to be considered."

I now knew he wasn't joking. And he is actually a very intelligent man. He truly believes that people should continue to eat animals and, in this case, continue to smoke cigarettes to keep these industries in business. It's somehow our responsibility to live less-than-healthy lives so our local meat, dairy, and tobacco farmers don't suffer.

His mention of the tobacco industry reminded me of something a nurse once told me that relates directly to the meat industry today. Sandy was a nurse in the late sixties in New York. She distinctly remembers the reps for Philip Morris and R. J. Reynolds visiting the hospital breakrooms, chitchatting with the personnel, and dropping off free cartons of cigarettes—by the case.

Big Tobacco knew that the best way to keep Americans lighting up was to entice the healthcare professionals with unlimited free cigarettes, so they stood as an example—silent salespeople—for every patient who was coming in with emphysema or early onset lung cancer. Smoking can't be bad for you if your healthcare professional smokes.

The FDA is doing the same thing for the meat, dairy, and egg industries through marketing and subsidies: make it possible to get more meat into more mouths more affordably so the sickness cycle continues. This is what we have become as consumers. The majority of Americans feel compelled to keep these industries profitable at the risk of their own health. It's insanity.

But the arguments for eating animals gets even more bizarre.

"Plants have feelings," a close friend said to me, trying to justify his choices for grilling burgers and hot dogs while I watched on. "I read this article about a study where they tested plants in a controlled setting. Every day three people would approach the plant and only one of the three would break off a leaf. After six months, the plant began to recognize the person who was breaking off the leaf."

He poked and prodded the perished pork.

According to what he heard, the plant leaned back and had a look of fear, or some such thing. He was telling me all this as he carefully turned the dead carcasses over with a spatula while my grilled portobello mushrooms, in the far back segregated corner of the grill, were beginning to burn. Two other friends walked up, beers in hand.

"Yeah, I heard this, too. How can you say you're vegan if you're actually killing something to eat it?" One friend chuckled, pointing at me with his Budweiser.

"Yeah, how can you?"

"If God didn't want us to eat animals, why did they make them out of meat?"

"Yeah . . . why? How?"

I was nudged. Poked and prodded.

"Vegans are such hypocrites."

"Well, Lindstrom? What do you have to say?"

Let's go back in time. The year was 1977. Elementary school. Dean De Falco was notorious for punching kids in the face, and I was told by Joey Leombrone that I going to be his next victim. Somehow, word got out at MacArthur Elementary School that today was my day. On October 11 at 2:35 p.m., I was going to be Dean's next victim. All day long, my ten-year-old heart pounded at the idea that I was the chosen one. I had never been in a fight before and didn't want to start now.

Throughout my elementary and middle school years, I was a scrawny kid who was more prey than predator; the art student who was writing or drawing while the bigger kids were tossing around a football, playing hockey, or punching each other in the face. I didn't even know how to punch, let alone avoid a punch. I'd say I blame my mom, but she'd easily knock any of these punks out with her wooden spoon if they so much as looked at me sideways.

But mom wasn't at school that day. Darn it.

The bell rang. I slowly walked outside under Binghamton's overcast skies. It was quiet. Too quiet. A group of kids appeared from out of nowhere and surrounded me, forming a perfect circle. The ring of death. Then, a small break in the circle opened for Dean to enter. He sauntered up and stood two inches away from me. I took it all in. His crew cut. His ten-year-old bulging biceps. His squinty eyes. (How does a ten-year-old have biceps?)

"You wouldn't punch a kid with glasses, would you?" I attempted, pointing at my new tortoise frames.

Dean pulled back and punched me. My glasses flew across the playground in slow motion as I fell to the ground. He climbed on top of me and punched me again and again as the kids cheered him on. For some reason, Captain and Tennille's "Muskrat Love" played in my head as I started to fade. All I could do was lie there on the pavement and take it.

But not anymore.

"Listen!" I started, confronting my friends at the barbecue. "Plants have *no* brain, *no* central nervous system, and *no* emotions. To compare cutting a head of lettuce to cutting the head off of a cow, or any other living being, is the most asinine thing any of you could ever say. When you clip parsley from your garden do you hear a scream? Would you bring your kids to a slaughterhouse or a farmers' market? Well?" I gave them all a Dean De Falco squint as I aggressively took a bite of a baby carrot dripping with hummus. Oh, yes, they did not know who they were dealing with.

"How can you *begin* to compare plants with frightened animals, cornered in their pen, grabbed by their hind legs and pulled from their family, just to have their throat slit or a nail gun shot into their heads? Or, worse. Dropped into a vat of boiling water while they are still alive. These sentient beings have feelings and souls and *don't* deserve to die for your taste buds. There are alternatives to killing animals for food. If I put a live rabbit and an apple in front of you and asked you to cut one up into bite-sized pieces, which would you choose?" I punctuated this last part in my best Steve McQueen impression. "Which. Would. You. Choose?"

Mic drop.

I grabbed the spatula and held it up to make my last remark.

"Now give me my mushroom. It's burning."

Still my all-time favorite animal eating–defensive comment is "If we didn't eat animals, what would happen to all the cows and chickens and pigs? Wouldn't they overpopulate and take over the world?" As if a world full of chickens were somehow going to manifest itself into "The Planet of the Chickens." A society where eighteen-inch-tall birds take over the world.

"Get your hands off me, you filthy chicken."

What these omnivores don't understand is that these animals, farm animals for simplification, are specifically being *bred* to be eaten and taken advantage of. These animals are born and raised to be killed. The more the demand for steak, the more cattle will be raised. The more hipsters cry for their bacon, the more pigs will be bred. The more Super Bowl–watching crowds eat chicken wings, the more chickens will be hatched. Stop the demand, and, eventually, the supply will stop, too. It's that simple. Furthermore, the three animals in the world to *not* be terrified of, *ever*, would probably be cows, chickens, and pigs.

If you think your own actions won't make a difference, imagine a line of dominoes, and the first domino is "going vegan." Now, be vegan. Tap that first domino and see what happens. The slightest ripple in the ocean becomes a massive wave on the shore.

The world needs more vegans. Vegans are making such incredible strides in the vegan and plant-based movement that soon omnivores are going to choose to eat meat simply out of anger, spite, and revenge.

> *The time will come when men such as I will look upon the*
> *murder of animals as they now look upon the murder of men.*
> *—Leonardo Da Vinci*

A few years back, a *Time Magazine* headline read: "Teen Found a Chicken Organ in His KFC Order." This is one of those many instances where being vegan truly felt right, knowing this would never happen to me. However, I did have to laugh thinking about this kid, and probably thousands more around the world, who find a body part in their fast food lunch or dinner order that, literally, is already comprised of body parts.

There was also that poor woman who was horrified at finding a chicken foot shrink-wrapped in the chicken breast packaging at her local grocer. That shrink-wrapped packaging that keeps body parts fresh long enough to bring home in time to cook to a temperature where it is safe enough to consume. For some reason, she was shocked to find that the very same package that contained body parts contained body parts.

This disconnect still baffles me, and it's happening thousands of times a day.

cog·ni·tive dis·so·nance [*noun*]: the state of having inconsistent thoughts, beliefs, or attitudes, especially as relating to behavioral decisions and attitude change.

Separating what is truth from what you want to believe. An example might be the guilt someone feels when eating a Cinnabon while on a diet. They know they shouldn't be eating it, but they like sweets. Two values—health and sweets—in conflict, creating a feeling of guilt.

Another example might be when people who enjoy eating meat are presented with imagery, or *facts,* about the known cruelty and obvious suffering of animals that colludes with their innate sense of compassion. This is a conflicting set of values—eating meat, and being compassionate; these emotions cannot coexist.

No matter what anyone tells you, you cannot truly be an animal lover and not be vegan.

This cognitive dissonance happens every day in society. Consider another poor, unfortunate, unsuspecting young woman who found a fully fried chicken head among her . . . um, fried chicken body parts. Not sure what she was expecting when she ordered it, but the chances of finding a dead animal in your order of fried dead animal is pretty high. That's no Happy Meal, especially for the animal.

That other victim, as reported in that *Time Magazine* article about KFC, said he eventually heard from a company official who assured him that the organ was probably just a gizzard or kidney and was completely edible. Okay, that's gross. Still, the episode may deter him from visiting KFC again soon. "I'm probably just going to have to start packing my own meals, making my own sandwiches," he said.

I am fairly confident his own sandwiches will have a 100 percent chance of containing dead animal.

If you don't want to be beaten, imprisoned, mutilated, killed,
or tortured, then you shouldn't condone such behavior towards
anyone, be they human or not.
—Moby

I recently reconnected with a high school friend of mine whom I hadn't been in touch with since John Cougar Mellencamp was just John Cougar and E. T. was trying to phone home on the new cellular radio telephone that was the size of a brick.

Matt was an outgoing and charismatic photographer in high school and a dynamic personality. His talent behind the lens became a career for him as a jet-setting, world traveling shutterbug for *Condé Nast Traveler*. His exploits, and his blog, eventually landed him a TV show that provided the platform for him to explore the finer things in life. From clothing to wine; from cars to food. And most of the time, the food featured was meat.

Lately, his full-time job with *Condé Nast Traveler* sends him to unbelievably exotic locations around the globe, and Matt embeds himself fully into the local cultures, traditions, and flavors and then reports back through the magazine, website, social media, and his own blog. His globetrotting is expertly expressed through his beautiful photography and journaling.

I keep up with Matt's antics and reserve any comments each time he posts something that features yet another dead animal. (Save for the occasional sarcastic "Is that vegan?" comment that I post on the photo of a dead boar hanging in a European butcher's window.) Some of these critters he may have actually killed himself while on location during a pheasant hunt or a fly fishing expedition.

If Matt's not posting a photo of a designer watch, a million-dollar car, or an expertly prepared dry martini, he's posting a photo of meat. Whether it's bacon in Brooklyn, foie gras in France, or free-range beef at his farm in Upstate New York, he's as much a meat eater as anyone I've ever known; perhaps more.

While researching this book, I was curious about just how deep his love for meat went after seeing a photo he took of the inside of a meat locker in London with the caption, "The Greatest Job in the World." So I called him. He had just returned from a video shoot in Los Angeles, and I caught him on his way from JFK to his place in Williamsburg.

"Hey, Matt. It's Eric." I thought I'd cut right to the point. "I have a question for you: why do you love meat so much?"

He knows I am vegan, he knows I am outspoken about it, and he knew I was writing this book. He is, himself, one of the many who occasionally comments "bacon" on a photo I post, but I've never really confronted him about our differences. I have to admit I am always curious what reasons any omnivore has for eating meat in this day and age. Especially Matt. I pride myself in always finding a counterargument to make someone at least *consider* veganism, either for health reasons or on behalf of the animals. It doesn't always resonate, though.

"I just love animal proteins," Matt said, probably already planning some sort of meaty dinner for himself and his wife and daughter back home. To his credit, he does prepare the most amazing-looking meals. "Pork and beef are my favorites, but all fowl is game on. And, of course, nothing is more perfect than the egg."

It's at this point where I would usually come back with, "Aren't you the least bit remorseful about killing and eating innocent animals?" Or, "Do you know where eggs actually come from and how truly bad they are for you?"

But Matt kept going.

"I feel my best, stronger, leaner, and healthier when my diet is packed with animal protein. I don't know what it is. My blood type or what. You hear doctors talk about the significance of that. There has to be some physiological connection."

A few years ago, an article surfaced about how pancreatic cancer risk increases with every two strips of bacon you eat. Processed meats, including sausage, pepperoni, bacon, ham, smoked turkey, and hot dogs, often contain nitrates, which have been tied to cancer. Every vegan I knew was quoting this article and using it as another example of why a vegan diet is best for optimal health.

Processed and smoked meats are poison.

Meanwhile, a few months later an article with a completely *opposite* argument was published that claimed bacon as a regular or moderate part of one's diet naturally works to *lower* the body's blood pressure and blood sugar levels. The report went on to explain how it could help to prevent and/or alleviate the effects of diabetes, as well as heart disease, stroke, and a potential heart attack. Which, of course, goes against any rationale for going vegan for health reasons and is the exact reason Matt continues to eat whatever he wants without concern for his own well-being.

Processed and smoked meats are medicinal.

Knowing all this, perhaps Matt would respond better to an animal rights angle? He owns two dogs, after all, and has a heart (likely clogged up, but a heart nonetheless).

"Is there any animal you won't eat? I mean, seriously, I've seen you eat pretty much any and all living creatures at one point or another. What wouldn't Matt eat?"

He paused.

"I will not eat a dog." Another pause. "Well if my life depended on it I guess I would. Only after eating the cat."

I don't think he was kidding.

At this point I had to go at him with the strongest, and most undeniable, argument against choosing to eat animals. No one would argue that nearly any animal that eventually becomes food suffers. If he believes his dogs have feelings, then he has to believe other sentient beings have feelings, too.

"Do you ever stop to think about animals as sentient beings?" I asked, with as convincing a tone as I could. "That they *feel* pain and experience fear? That they suffer?"

Matt sighed and reflected for a moment.

"Listen, I love animals and have thoughtful, caring, sensitive relationships with them." *Here we go*, I thought, *he's going to use the word* humanely *any second now.* "I raised pigs to eat for seven years of my life and adored and admired them. They are smart, clever, discerning eaters, and I loved my time with them."

I actually didn't know this about him but was still waiting for "the word."

"That respect made it easier for me to care for them, give them a comfortable life, and then kill them humanely." There it was. "And eat them. *Nothing* goes to waste when you harvest a pig, and I loved them for that. I could not live without pork."

Well, actually, you could, I thought. But I was silent. I should have come back at that point with an argument about his use of the word *humanely* as it applied to killing any animal, but I knew Matt truly believed what he was saying. I knew he was speaking from a place of integrity, and nothing I would say after that would change his thinking. I had been there myself. I have eaten more than my share of animals. I used to think the exact same way Matt thinks. I was an omnivore. That was before I went vegan overnight on a bet.

One last attempt.

"What if someone challenged you to go vegan for thirty days, would you do it? For your daughter?" I asked, as I heard the sounds of Brooklyn in the background as Matt climbed out of the car. He was home and ready to hang up.

I think, from Matt's perspective, the conversation was over before it started.

"Why would I ever need to take that 'challenge' to prove *what* to myself or someone else? Listen, I know I could do it easily—I just *choose* not to. I like the variety in my diet and that does include vegetables, by the way. You're who you are, and I am who I am."

"You're an unapologetic omnivore, aren't you?"

"I am unapologetically an omnivore," he concluded. "I also subscribe to the philosophy that we humans, not unlike bears, are designed to be that way. Goodnight, Eric."

He hung up.

Every so often, but not *very* often, I come across someone who is the exact opposite of me in my thinking. Someone so steeped in speciesism while remaining steadfast in their personal beliefs. Someone I can still relate to and choose not to try to sway or convince otherwise. Someone whom I respect and admire for their personal accomplishments in life as well as their true honesty.

Matt is one of these people who, in my book, gets away with murder.

20

DEFENDING VEGANISM

First they ignore you, then they ridicule you,
then they fight you, and then you win.
—*Mahatma Gandhi*

"I've never eaten vegan food before," numerous well-meaning omnivore friends have whispered to me at vegan restaurants, as if it's some sort of a *stretch* to eat vegan food. They lean in, as if it's some sort of a confession.

They peer at me from across the booth. A dark latticed screen blurs their face. Chanting monks can be heard in the distance.

"Forgive me, Father, for I have sinned. It has been three hours since I last ate an animal. I've been cooking bacon and eggs nearly every morning this month, and I drooled over a photo of a beef taco."

"And, how do you feel about this, my son?"

"I felt wonderful until I had to go to dinner with a *vegan*."

"I see."

"Oh, and, Father, I lied to a cop when he asked if I knew how fast I was driving. I knew."

"And how did *that* make you feel?"

"Fine. I mean, lying is one thing, and, honestly, I don't think I was doing fifty in a thirty, but ordering a vegan meal is something I am completely uncomfortable with. I am fearful of being judged, Father. I just don't know what to do. Do I dare order the cheeseburger? For these and all the sins of my past life, I ask pardon of God, penance, and absolution from you, Father."

"I see. Say ten Kale Marys and ten How's Your Fathers for your penance. And just order the pasta with vegetables, and a side salad with oil and vinegar, for God's sake. It's really not that difficult."

My friends carefully watch my every move whenever we go out to eat at nonvegan restaurants. Curiously follow my eyes around the menu to see how I skillfully construct an actual meal out of three sides, rice, and some vegetables.

How can someone survive only eating plants? they think. *Isn't that how rabbits eat?*

Whenever someone tells me they've never eaten vegan food, I'll always answer with, "So, you've never eaten peanut butter and jelly sandwiches, pasta, rice, fruits and vegetables, oatmeal, guacamole, beans, hummus, or Oreo cookies?"

Then I come at them with the big guns. The mother of all vegan foods that everyone has had in their lives. "Or french fries? You've never eaten french fries?"

Sometimes this response puts them somewhat on the defensive. Of course they've eaten french fries before. Of course they've had a salad as a side. Or vegetable soup. I know what they mean when they say they've never eaten "vegan food" before.

"You *know* what I mean," they huff and proceed to order a double bacon cheeseburger with bleu cheese just to spite me.

Incredibly, you are going to find yourself defending compassionate living and your vegan diet. Society has been so ingrained for so long about the virtues and traditions of eating meat, the health "advantages" of drinking milk, and the "it doesn't hurt the chicken to take their eggs" ideology, that you find yourself up against the wall more often than not.

People will come at you from all sides with their defense of their own actions. Actions they support by validating their diet and lifestyle as "their choice," not once stopping to consider the choice or the feelings of animals. They will tell you about how early humans were the healthiest and that a Paleo Diet is best for losing weight and feeling great. Of course, what they forget to realize is that cavemen only lived to the ripe old age of thirty-five. Even if a Neanderthal man fed on carcasses of a Mastodon, and new evidence showed they also dined on each other, it was never their primary source of food.

I once posted an article about the awful conditions at a South Carolina pig farm. The accompanying video showed torture and animal cruelty that eventually shut this particular farm down until they could implement stricter and safer practices. To this day, they are still closed. The first comment from a meat-eating friend read: "Thanks! Now I'm going to order more pepperoni and sausage on my pizza tonight." People are like this.

When faced with actual compassion and ethical decisions, they recoil and attack with the one thing they are familiar with: eating animals. Whether they care to admit it, they feel guilt on some deep level for what they're doing, or supporting; otherwise they wouldn't feel the need to defend themselves.

Every animal on the planet has as much a right to live as any human. We share the air and earth with all creatures—two-legged, four-legged, eight-legged, winged, and finned. *Animals deserve better.*

Not a single attempt at marketing meat as "humanely slaughtered," or any of the other yuppie terms that have been invented since I wrote this paragraph, changes the fact that the animals are killed against their will at the end. If you're at all in doubt, there are plenty of videos online of pigs scattering in fear as the farmer decides which one is to be chosen. Pigs are smarter, and more social, than dogs, and I don't think anyone would label a dog "humanely killed" if its throat were slit and its head were pulled through an aluminum funnel.

In fact, it's against the law.

There's another video of two cows standing in line on their way to be slaughtered. Once one cow walks through the metal gate, the other cow backs up in actual fear. She knows exactly what's happening on the other side of the wall, and she knows she is next.

I've also known quite a few vegetarians over the years, including Jen when we first met, who have to deal with this after becoming vegan. (By the way, vegetarians become vegan when they grow up.) These vegetarians take that last important step for the animals and commit to a vegan lifestyle. And yet, they are suddenly ostracized by and questioned about their choices. While I have my own opinion about vegetarians' weakness for cheese and eggs, I do sympathize with them when they are subjected to the same level of scrutiny as vegans even when they used to be vegetarians.

Vegetarians (who are not yet vegan) usually don't have to put up with much. In fact, most responses to their vegetarianism are "That's nice." But as soon as they go vegan, the nutritional advice begins, and in some instances, the hate starts rolling in. It's as if all of society is truly against admitting certain animals have a right to live.

> *The greatness of a nation and its moral progress can be judged by the way its animals are treated.*
> — *Mahatma Gandhi*

Out of sheer curiosity, I tuned in to a live Periscope broadcast of a tour of an Upstate New York foie gras farm. The broadcast was hosted by a reputable media outlet, and the Hudson Valley Foie Gras Ducks Products farm boasted throughout the online broadcast about the "ethical and humane treatment" of their waterfowls. During the tour, they reported that in order to produce foie gras, they replicate the natural gorging process of the birds by forcing a feeding tube directly down the duck's throat and gorging them with feed until their liver explodes. Of course, they didn't say it in these words. They claimed that this special hand-feeding process optimizes what "nature gives us" and that they are able to produce high quality ducks. The result? A "luxurious foie gras that is at once velvety and umami." They are also simultaneously producing a terrified and tortured dead duck.

Doesn't that sound fancy? *So French.*

During the live broadcast, as the owner of the farm led the camera through the darkened facility, you could actually see the ducks fleeing, in terror, each time any humans got too close. They are well aware of their fate and have to live this stressful existence for their entire shortened lives. Try this same live walking tour concept at any animal sanctuary, and you'll immediately see my point.

According to The Bible, it is okay to eat animals, and so a few friends, who probably would explode into an instant fireball if they ever set foot in a church, use *this* as an excuse. The Bible also says you can keep slaves, shouldn't eat fat, and shouldn't be gay. Or, if you find that the people in the city you're visiting worship another god, you have to kill them all. Not nice, Bible. Also, since when is The Bible a dining guide?

"My body requires meat, and I can't get enough [insert nutrient or protein here] on a vegan diet. I tried." Any excuse to not commit.

When I first went vegan, I asked a young woman who was *raw* vegan the very same question: "So, what do you do about protein?"

She said, "I never think about it."

This was six years ago. I haven't thought about my protein ever since.

Everything you need to live a (very) long and healthy life can be gotten from a plant-based diet. In fact, a whole-food, plant-based diet, the healthiest diet on the planet, is one that has been proven to help avoid or cure certain cancer, diabetes, osteoporosis, and the number one killer of adults in the US, heart disease. In his landmark book *Prevent and Reverse Heart Disease*, Dr. Caldwell Esselstyn argues that coronary artery disease is preventable, even after its effects are underway, with little use of drugs or expensive medical equipment. The answer lies in nutrition, specifically plant-based nutrition.

> *Big Meat and Big Pharma don't want you to know this.*
> *I can't think of anything better in the world to be but a vegan.*
> —*Alicia Silverstone*

I think one of the more interesting aspects about being vegan is the reaction you'll get from friends and family members who knew you as an omnivore their entire lives. They will inevitably think you're going through a phase and wonder when you plan on returning to your meat-eating ways. They'll be oddly inquisitive about what you eat and what it contains.

The common comment "You eat *that*? What's in it anyway?" is uttered anytime anyone sees you order, make, or offer them vegan food.

My own mother is guilty of this. If I ask her to try vegan cheese, for example, she will always ask, *what's in it anyway?* As if the vegan version of food has its own agenda or is conspiracy-laden. That vegan food is, for whatever reason, terrible for your health and you should question every ingredient. They'll ask *you* to question every ingredient. Where this becomes particularly hilarious to me is that these very same people never *once* asked me what was in *anything* I ate when I was an omnivore. *Ever.*

And if you knew what was actually *in* your bacon cheeseburger and the process involved in getting it to your plate, you'd go vegan.

Exhibit A: VioLife vegan cheese. VioLife is the vegan cheese company that started in Greece, swept across Europe and Asia, and recently came ashore to the United States. They set the standard for what vegan cheese should look and taste like, and I personally believe they may be responsible for thousands of vegetarians finally becoming vegan.

VioLife vegan slices (mushroom flavor) ingredients include water, coconut oil, modified starch, sea salt, dried mushrooms, vegan flavors (spices), citric acid, and b-Carotene. Compare this to a leading "gourmet" dairy cheese slice's (natural) ingredients: milk, whey, milk protein concentrate, sodium citrate, calcium phosphate, whey protein concentrate, salt, lactic acid, sorbic acid, cheese culture, paprika, enzymes, and Vitamin D3.

Of course, you have to bear in mind that with the top ingredient being milk in all dairy cheeses, you also get these delicious added ingredients not listed on the label and at no additional charge: pus, blood, bacteria, rennet (stomach lining), morphine, codeine, artery-clogging saturated fats, high bad cholesterol—and, for added palatability, rape, torture, and murder.

I'd rather choose the vegan version of anything that tastes as good as its nonvegan counterpart.

Exhibit B: Vegan cupcakes. While celebrating a coworker's birthday at work one day, I brought my own vegan cupcakes in addition to the regular cake and ice cream. My cupcakes looked, and tasted, exactly like "normal" cupcakes. Half their height of frosting rested precariously over a soft, tasty vanilla cake in a wax paper liner.

You've seen cupcakes before.

One coworker was late to the party, and she was disappointed to find out that the cake was gone. I offered her a cupcake.

"Is it vegan?" she asked, nose pinched and eyes squinting, already knowing the answer, since it was *I* who was offering it to her.

"Yes, and it's delicious."

"Ew. No, thanks, I'll pass."

Pass on a cupcake because it's vegan? As if eggs are the primary, and sought-after, taste that people seek in their cupcakes. Or that frosting can only be made with a pound of butter and heavy cream? Her refusal to eat one only meant there were more for me.

"You *can* eat that, you *choose* not to," my brother-in-law said to me about a Buffalo wing dip my mother made one Christmas. I had just become vegan earlier that year, and he, among countless others, assumed it was a passing fad or some "diet" I was trying out to shed some pounds. When the dip was offered to me, I responded immediately: "Thanks, but I can't eat that." Which, as David then pointed out in his own words, was not true. I *could* have, but I chose not to. I reminded him that, years earlier, he himself had been vegetarian, and it wouldn't have crossed my mind to offer him meat, since he certainly wouldn't have eaten it. There have been hundreds of dishes I've passed since going vegan, and every day that I am still vegan, I am more and more sure of my decision. Going vegan was the single most important decision of my life, and one that I know I will hold onto forever.

Going vegan is a commitment. You're probably going to lose some friends after transitioning, but you're going to pick up new (better) friends along the way, as well as a *lot* of friends in the animal kingdom.

A vegan friend of mine recently told me about a situation she was dealing with regarding her four-year-old daughter's daycare. The well-respected facility was conducting a fundraiser to raise money to expand their main building. Aside from (nonvegan) bake sales throughout the year, they launched a "paver dedication program" where families could purchase a sidewalk brick and have their family name, dog name, company name, favorite quote, or saying etched into a twelve-by-twelve paver as a permanent part of the walkway. My friend's daughter had a great idea for the paver. They filled out the form, made their check out for $250, and wrote neatly on the page the letters GO VEGAN. They dropped it at the front desk.

"They called me at home that night and left a message," she told me over coffee. "I called them back to find out they rejected Maggie's paver."

"They rejected the phrase *Go Vegan*?"

"Yeah. They said they had a policy about committing an agenda to the sidewalk and felt the phrase was too heavy-handed, so we filled out another form that said: LOVE ANIMALS. DON'T EAT THEM. Amazingly, they turned that down, too." She laughed.

"They really are opposed to animals at this daycare, aren't they?" I asked.

"So, we tried once more and sent in THOU SHALT NOT KILL as a joke, and they accepted it," she said. "We're now the religious freaks instead of the vegan weirdos."

> *We are, quite literally, gambling with the future*
> *of our planet—for the sake of hamburgers.*
> *—Peter Singer*

"What would you like for your protein?" The server asked me after taking my order at a well-known fast casual restaurant.

In her mind, she was probably working her way around the plate and trying to be helpful by "filling in the blanks" left by my special order and vegan diet. The omnivores at my table, on the other hand, had ordered "complete meals" that consisted of starch (most likely potatoes), some vegetables (almost always swimming in melted cheese sauce), and "the protein," in this case, chicken.

"What do you mean, 'what do I want for my protein?' There's protein in all of what I just ordered," I answered, not at all trying to be difficult. I wanted to point out that protein comes in *all* foods.

In some cases, defending veganism is as simple as educating those around you about what it means to leave meat off your plate. In this instance, I had ordered garlic olive oil linguine that came topped with broccoli, zucchini, and cherry tomatoes—the vegetables the kitchen had on hand. I also ordered a side salad with oil and vinegar dressing.

This meal came complete "with protein." There were approximately 5 g of protein in the pasta, 6.5 g in the broccoli, 4.5 g in the zucchini, and 3 g in the tomatoes. Add another 3 g for the garlic and other greens. This particular vegan meal had 21 g of protein. A full third of one day's recommended protein requirement with no cholesterol, abundant burnable calories, and very little fat. There is *literally* no reason to eat animals for protein.

I use the word *literally* very sparingly.

When you consider that all of the planet's largest animals are actually *herbivores*, there really is no longer a valid health argument against going vegan.

The concept that you are not ingesting rotting flesh sort of sums it up for me.
—Bryan Adams

For every person I know who is opposed to being vegan, there are just as many who are curious and who welcome conversations about being vegan. One friend in particular, Sly, has started practicing "Meatless Mondays" at his office in Houston. He and a coworker take this one day per week to eat no meat. It's a great start.

I've had Sly over for dinner a few times, and he remains the most open-minded and inquisitive about being vegan. The vegan fried chickenless strips, dipped in Ranch dressing, and cheezy soyrizo quesadillas keep him coming back. One year, we met up with him in Phoenix and asked him to join us at the Green New American Vegetarian (Vegan) restaurant in Tempe (not to be confused with tempeh, which is made from whole soybeans and is thus a less processed version of tofu).

Chef Damon Brasch has perfected fast casual vegan food to such an extent that if you bring an omnivore there to eat, which we did, they wouldn't know they weren't eating meat or consuming dairy. In a good way. Buffalo wings, spinach fundido, chili fries, Thai peanut rice bowls, and one other item that keeps the vegans, and the omnivores, coming back.

"This is Sly's first time to Green. What should he order?" I asked the tattooed cashier at the front counter, knowing full well what she was going to say. I had already ordered a milkshake, chili fries with cheese, and wings. "He's not vegan, but he's very open-minded about it all," I added.

She sized Sly up and down. He's a big man.

"The Big Wac," she said, nodding, without hesitation.

"The. Big. Wac," I repeated, for drama. Whenever I repeat anything for "drama," I use one word sentences. An old advertising trick.

The Big Wac is just what it sounds like: a vegan version of the burger that made the scary, kid-killing clown famous. The Big Wac is two hand-packed vegan patties, special sauce, lettuce, cheese, pickles, onions on a sesame seed bun. Sound familiar?

We sat at an empty booth and started to dig into my wings and fries while we waited for the Big Wac attack. Sly grew up in nearby Phoenix and had never been to Green—and why would he? He eats meat, and he eats at restaurants that serve meat. He has limited opportunities to try new things and, until that very moment, thought vegan food was boring and tasteless. Omnivores are so set in their ways that it's difficult for them to accept that vegan food can be at all satisfying or sinful. The Big Wac, washed down with a vanilla milkshake, is both.

"Satisfying. Sinful," Sly said after taking just one bite of the burger. Some special sauce found its way into his beard. "Really great."

Friends like Sly, and people who are generally adventurous in life, will embrace your veganism. When they take chances, they'll be surprised at how great vegan food is.

> *Why are vegans made fun of while the inhumane factory farming process regards animals and the natural world merely as commodities to be exploited for profit?*
> *—Ellen Page*

By now you know that vegans are so accustomed to defending themselves and their lifestyles that they've literally crafted a counterpoint to every point made by argumentative animal eaters. The vegan vs. meat eater debate is endless and usually goes something like this:

"Man evolved to eat meat," says the animal eater.

"Actually, from an optimal health perspective and for the sake of the planet's health, man is evolving *away* from eating meat," replies the tofu muncher, while munching on tofu.

"Our teeth are suited for eating meat."

"Technically, human canines are neither elongated nor sharp and are better equipped for eating fruits, vegetables, and grains. We chew side to side, not straight up and down. When was the last time you tore fur-covered flesh off of a dead animal, and when was the last time you ate an apple?"

"Well, meat is delicious."

"If you think about it, the flavors you are experiencing are introduced through *vegan* spices and marinades. Very few meats are 'delicious' without vegan intervention."

"Animals don't have feelings."

"Kick your dog in the head and then get back to me on this one. Or don't, since I'm sure you get my point without having to actually kick your dog."

"Plants have feelings, though."

"No, they don't. No central nervous system. No brain. No feelings. Some plants respond to stimuli, but they do not feel pain. We went over this."

"My decision to eat meat is a personal decision. It's my choice."

"You're saying the billions of animals needlessly slaughtered every year have no say in their own lives? *They* have no choice?"

"But, where would I get my protein?"

"The same place your protein gets *its* protein. Plants are abundant in protein. You don't need to think about protein as a food group, but, if you must, think about tofu, nondairy milks, and plant-based meat substitutes. Navy beans have as much protein as chicken per serving. This is just another excuse."

"If we didn't eat the animals, they would overpopulate the planet."

"Not true. The animals you are most likely referring to are actually being *bred* to be eaten. Stop the demand, and then supply will stop, too. Besides, farm animals already outnumber humans by a ratio of 65:1 so we are the minority already and at risk of being attacked. By cows, pigs, and chickens."

"Cows need to be milked in order to stay healthy."

"Cows lactate to provide milk to their offspring, which are baby cows, not humans. Milking cows are either being artificially inseminated, pregnant, having their newborn stolen from them, or being milked while lactating. If you stopped this cycle, you'd stop the need to milk cows in the first place. Let the calves have their milk."

"Vegan food is too expensive, and the diet is for the elite."

"Compare the price of meat and other animal products against the price of vegetables and grains, and you'll find that vegetables and grains are always more affordable. And the government artificially lowers the price of animal foods by subsidizing "feed" crops. Beans and rice are not the food of kings and queens. Give peas a chance."

"If everyone became vegan, farmers would suffer."

"Over time, farms that produce meat would be as profitable producing fruits, vegetables, and grains. An argument for eating animals so a farmer in Nebraska can stay in business is a very strange argument, unless you happen to be that farmer living in Nebraska."

"The Bible says to eat meat."

"The Bible was published in the year 96 AD. The Bible also says if a woman breaks up a fight, you can cut off her hand. Also, that you can purchase slaves from any foreigners among us. And, according to The Bible, kids are thrown into that slave deal for free. Additionally, the punishment for rape is marrying the victim. This is the same Bible that mentions the walking dead, born from a virgin. Just saying."

"Chorizo."

"Soyrizo."

"Cheese."

"Vegan cheese."

"No one can be 100 percent vegan, so why bother?"

"This is true, but *everyone* can try 100 percent of the time."

"Bacon."

The *real* question meat eaters need to ask themselves is why they would argue against any individual trying to make a positive change for themselves, the planet, and for the animals.

> *Being vegan just gives you such great karma.*
> —*Alicia Silverstone*

Omnivores, beware. We are coming. Vegans are building a brigade. Our numbers are increasing nationally, and internationally, every day.

A regiment of herbivores is forming. An advanced human who can survive purely on plant-based foods. This contingent is growing in size and in strength. We soon will take over your grocery stores, your farmer's markets, your fast food restaurants, and your dinner tables. You won't see us coming. There will be little warning. But we are there. Hiding. Behind the bushes (that we are nourished by). Plotting this initiative at vegan potlucks and dishes-to-pass.

We are peaceful in our approach. Slowly educating the masses. Eliminating the enemies. Removing the Paula Deens and replacing them with the Jason Wrobels. Resistance is futile. Eventually, each one of you will eat a salad. Each one of you will enjoy kale—that has been simply steamed, with some chopped-up garlic.

You will eat tofu and love it. You will suddenly feel better. You will lose weight. You will change the course of your current downward spiral in your health. And you, too, shall become strong. Strong enough to join the Vegan Brigade. We are always recruiting.

And just when you think that we cannot win, that our numbers simply aren't strong enough, that our bodies aren't fit enough, that we don't get enough protein, that we're weakened by the lack of B12 in our scrawny bodies, it is then that you will be reminded . . .

We have the rest of the animal kingdom on our side.

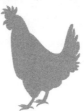

21

CRAVINGS, VEGAN POTLUCKS, AND THE HOLIDAYS

Do not confuse your cravings with your needs.
—Renji George

I met this woman who was "vegan" at one point in her life but who started eating meat again because, according to her, "the platter of chicken was passed under my nose, and my body told me I needed it." My own nutritionist, who was once vegan, then vegetarian, and now omnivore, said she literally started drooling as she passed the meat counter at our local grocery store. She stands by the belief that some humans do, in fact, require meat for optimal health.

So, for future reference, an easy way "out" of being vegan is to simply give in to cravings and just start eating meat again. If you decide that veganism isn't for you, by all means, stop being vegan. Listen to your body and make the choice to start eating meat again—or, be strong and think about the animals.

Of course, once you have *fully* transitioned to being vegan in the truest sense of the word, there will no longer be such a thing as "craving meat." It will be impossible to ever imagine bringing harm to or consuming an animal, under any and every circumstance. The idea of tearing meat off a bone that once belonged to an innocent animal, or chewing on a burger that contains any number of animal parts, makes me sick to my stomach. I feel the same way about dairy milk.

Early on in my journey, I admitted to cravings. I looked longingly at the basket of wings being passed around or the steak being brushed on the grill. I can admit that now. However, after years of being vegan and "making the connection," it's literally impossible for me to crave meat, dairy, or eggs. My mind and my body won't let me.

There have been numerous high-profile "vegans" who have made the claim that their bodies suddenly requested meat—that they woke up omnivore. They felt weak or weakened and began to bring meat, usually starting with some type of fish, back into their diets. These celebrities built immense social media followings and massive fan bases, only to one day "come out" and confess that they'd started eating bison (albeit grass-fed, free-range bison) or that they were sneaking into their basement and eating wild-caught salmon.

These people were never *really* vegan. They were at most *plant-based*. They did, however, get some nice book deals out of their experience. Once a vegan, always a vegan.

True vegans cannot go back. They know too much.

The story of one such very famous "vegan" who later came out as a closeted omnivore received national news exposure. According to an interview on CBS, she "revealed the dark underbelly of veganism." What she did bring to light was something known as orthorexia, a real condition that includes symptoms of *obsessive* behavior in pursuit of an overly healthy diet. Orthorexia sufferers often display signs and symptoms of anxiety disorders that frequently co-occur with anorexia nervosa or other eating disorders. You can take being healthy, skinny, and vegan too far, and she took it too far and had to get a handle on her health again. Unfortunately, she chose an omnivore diet to get there.

Some vegans are presented with the bizarre scenario of being stranded on a deserted island and left to die. Would they eat the animals on the island to survive, thereby relinquishing their vegan beliefs?

The short answer to this is that if there are animals thriving on the island, there is also likely plant-based food and fresh water—enough for humans to survive on. The longer answer is that vegans would, begrudgingly, do whatever they needed to do to survive. This same scenario comes into play for these former vegans who claim their bodies need animal protein to survive. Of course, this isn't true. If they were the ones stranded on a deserted island and could only live off fruits and vegetables, they would be in the best shape of their lives, living longer without heart disease, diabetes, obesity, and certain types of cancer, all while soaking up unlimited amounts of Vitamin D.

Where do I sign up?

Becoming vegan is the most important and direct change we can immediately make to save the planet and its species.
—*Chris Hedges*

But what about medications or vaccines? All of which have either been tested on animals or require some level of animal involvement? Most vegans would take a pill to live.

Every so often, I find out about something that is so outrageous and disgusting, I have to stop everything I'm doing to appreciate the fact that I'm vegan. The use of beaver anal sac excretions in my morning cereal to give it that yummy "beaver-approved" natural vanilla flavoring was one of these things I never could have imagined.

Amazingly, the anal sac issue pales by comparison to what I found out about the prescription drug *Premarin*, used to treat hot flashes, irritation, and other symptoms of menopause. Listen, I get it, menopause is a very uncomfortable time for women. But any amount of discomfort cannot compare to the practice of impregnating horses, limiting their water intake *and* movement, collecting their urine for use in the drug, and then killing their offspring. In some cases, the "lucky" foals get to live so they can lead the same enslaved lives as their mother.

This is where this drug Premarin comes from. The word *mare* is in their clever brand name, and the drug company Pfizer still offers it today, along with countless other prescription medications that either abuse or use animals.

Any form of animal abuse is bad, and I am often criticized for singling out what abuse I think is "worse" than others. The fact that it is legal to eat your own cat or dog in forty-three United States disgusts me, but, technically, it's no worse than the billions of animals that are mistreated and killed for food around the world. What gets me about Premarin is that there are options that do not involve animal secretions or animal testing. In fact, these options simply involve changing your diet. To vegan.

Nearly all symptoms of menopause can be controlled by going vegan. A high intake of phytoestrogens is thought to explain why hot flashes and other menopausal symptoms rarely occur in populations consuming a predominantly plant-based diet. Increased intake of phytoestrogens by consuming more soy milk, linseed, tofu, tempeh, miso, pumpkin seeds, sesame seeds, sunflower seeds, celery, rhubarb, and green beans will help with menopause.

I know, I know—going vegan is drastic, whereas paying someone else to rape and enslave a beautiful mare, dehydrate her, collect her urine while she is pregnant, and subsequently kill her useless offspring isn't.

I've said it once before and I will say it again: when it comes to Big Pharma, Pfuck Pfizer.

So, what about vaccines?

In 2015, Marin County, California, home to rich white people and yoga studios, had a measles outbreak. This active and healthy county nestled along the Pacific Ocean just north of San Francisco became the epicenter of a nationwide antivax movement, a trend that goes back over a decade and has been largely to blame for California's ongoing measles outbreaks that put health officials and parents on edge.

Measles, polio, smallpox, mumps, and a variety of other debilitating diseases are guarded against through vaccinations usually given to infants before they turn three. In fact, polio has been almost completely wiped off the planet because of vaccines.

These same entitled and privileged people bring their unvaccinated children to potlucks, risking the lives of other younger children who cannot be vaccinated because they are either too young or have a low immunity, making immunization risky. Of course, these very same people are likely vaccinated, since their parents most likely aren't trend-following lunatics who believe that vaccines cause autism or are part of some other government conspiracy to pollute our population.

No vaccines are vegan. In fact, no medications are. At some point, some level of animal testing has taken place; the FDA requires it. As a result, some vegans I know are antivaxxers because vaccines are not vegan.

When all of this came into clear focus for us, our second baby had already been born. Newborns cannot be vaccinated, and we couldn't risk our little one being exposed. So, we had to avoid vegan events for a full year until she could be protected from the antivaxxers' children.

This inspired Jen to write this editorial, which captures exactly my feelings on all of this:

> Most vegans I know are introspective and give deep, meaningful thought to how their actions and choices affect others and our planet. Most vegans I know think critically about social, political, and economic disparities. Most vegans I know are trying to live an ethical and moral life and help others along the way. Most vegans I know are concerned about the health and well-being of themselves and their loved ones. Most vegans I know are nonviolent folks who wouldn't want to permanently and severely damage or kill other people, including innocent babies.
>
> Most vegans I know wouldn't drink and drive, endangering their lives and others, even though it's their personal choice to drink. Most vegans I know have a visceral reaction to the unnecessary suffering of animals and also don't like the thought of seeing their fellow humans suffer. Most vegans I know wouldn't visit an oncology ward with even a head cold, knowing a simple cold to someone with a compromised immune system could give them pneumonia. Most vegans I know don't exercise their constitutional right to bear arms, thereby making it impossible for them to accidentally shoot other people, even though it would be their personal choice to own a gun. Most vegans I know are loving and compassionate, and I'm fortunate to have them in my life.

And yet, it is indisputably the fault of anti-vaxxers that we are seeing a serious, highly contagious, and potentially deadly disease reemerge in this country of wealth and privilege and education and freedom. Most vegans I know—my friends—wouldn't want my baby to suffer brain damage or blindness or deafness—or even death. Yet their very presence in a room with my daughter could kill her. Most vegans I know want to do the right thing for themselves, their families, their friends, and for the good of public health.

Most vegans I know strive for an organic lifestyle free of toxins, yet most vegans I know breathe air (polluted with toxins), drink water (polluted with sterilizing chemicals), eat out at non-organic restaurants, touch plastics, wear non-organic cotton, buy clothes, and use iPhones, droids, and computers made halfway around the world in sweatshops. Most vegans I know use unsustainable energy, drive cars, fly in airplanes, and generally leave a carbon footprint every day despite recycling efforts, water conservation, and being vegan. Most vegans I know believe in the science of climate change, the science of nutrition, and science in general, but choose to deny the science of vaccines. Most vegans I know aren't perfect people, but they're doing the best they can.

And some vegans choose not to vaccinate for vegan reasons, while knowing that the vaccines may actually be beneficial. We vaccinate.

> *We choose to eat meat and have therefore built*
> *slaughterhouses for the animals and hospitals for us.*
> *—Akbarali Jetha*

Most vegans want to be healthier. However, they *are* only human after all and may find themselves really experiencing meat cravings. This is not a sin, and there is an answer. Look to seitan. Feeling naughty and want a grilled Reuben? Seitan is the answer. Praying that there will, one day, be a meat replacement that feels, tastes, cooks, and looks like meat? All Hail Seitan.

Seitan, the vegan "wheat meat," is the amazing result of simmering wheat gluten, the stretchy substance that gives dough and bread its texture, with flavored water and spices to create a loaf of vital wheat gluten or "wheat meat." Sort of like a very dense loaf of bread that is savory and can be sliced and diced and eaten like meat. Seitan truly takes on the personality of meat and is the basis of many of the faux meats on the market. When vital wheat gluten is used as an ingredient in sausage, patties, or shreds, you'll immediately be fooled into thinking you're no longer vegan.

Even though you are.

Some vegans can't stomach seitan because its taste and texture is frequently too real for their comfort level. I happen to love it and am lucky enough to actually have a friend who operates a successful seitan business.

"Little did I know, when I started my vegan food business in Ithaca twenty-four years ago, that Susie's Seitan would become a household name," Susie said to me over a spicy seitan sandwich. "I thought they would be famous just in Ithaca, of course. Now my products are everywhere. Seitan is such a versatile food, and there are so many things you can make with it. During my festival days working food stands and food trucks, I made gyros, burritos, Cuban sandwiches, and so on and so forth."

Susie is so adept at making seitan, and her products are so well known and loved that the majority of people actually think her real name is Susie Seitan. (Come to think of it, that might actually be her name.)

While seitan may help ward off a craving, one really interesting dynamic of going vegan is how much your taste buds are going to change, in both directions.

Growing up, I used to eat all the popular sugary cereals while sitting in front of the TV with my little sister, watching *Little House on the Prairie*. Count Chocula, Frankenberry, Quisp, Cap'n Crunch, and my all-time favorite, Fruity Pebbles. These brightly-colored miniature pebbles of flavor rocked my mouth as often as my mom would allow. I'd polish off two bowls and then drink down the bowl full of brightly colored milk, ready to bounce off of every wall and drive my teachers crazy that day at West Middle School.

Well, as if the news were sent from heaven, I've found that Fruity Pebbles *are* vegan. (As are Cap'n Crunch, Reese's Puffs, Corn Pops, and countless others of these childhood favorites, though for the record, none of these are the least bit good for you, and the toys really suck.) I rushed to the store, drove home at a speed that risked a speeding ticket, tore open the box (did a quick check to see if there was a cheap toy in the bottom), poured a bowl, doused it in soy milk, closed my eyes, took one bite . . . and . . . almost threw up.

It tasted like paint. Or petroleum. Or some other toxic substance they use to lure and addict innocent little kids to sugary breakfast cereals. It didn't taste good at all, and it left a strange coating on my tongue that I had to scrape off with a toothbrush.

What did I learn? Well, first off, I think I got a little too excited about eating Fruity Pebbles, considering I was a forty-six-year-old man at the time; but, more important, after two years of being vegan, my taste buds had changed. Instead of laboratory-developed faux flavors and added chemicals that mimic "natural flavors," I actually now prefer natural flavors. As in, flavors from nature.

Fruit. *Ever hear of it?* Give me a bowl of cut-up bananas, grapes, apples, strawberries, and blueberries any day over a bowl of Fruity Pebbles. Trust me on this, you do *not* have to conduct this same cereal experiment for yourself. It will have the same unpleasant results.

The majority of vegans I've talked to have experienced the same reactions. Not necessarily to breakfast cereals, but to other foods they used to enjoy. Vegan taste buds, like vegans themselves, have evolved. People who once shied away from spinach now love it. So many vegans are in love with kale, while I'm pretty sure I can say with all confidence that meat eaters don't love kale.

The other day, I was talking to a teen vegan who had made his own decision to go vegan and was lucky enough to get the support of his entire family. He told me how great he felt and how much he enjoyed foods he wouldn't have even tried just a few years earlier.

"I hated tomatoes, onions, and bell peppers before," he said. "Like, I would even pick them out of my food; I hated them that much. Now I love them! It still shocks my mom when she sees me eating a tomato after years of dislike." He went on, "I find that raw veggies and fruits seem so much more flavorful and satisfying now. It's like I am fully experiencing the flavor now that I don't have meat and dairy polluting my body. I used to not like peppers as an omnivore, and now one of my favorites are raw peppers."

This dude was the same age that I was when I was eating three bowls of Fruity Pebbles in my Spider-Man pajamas. You cannot be too young or too old to appreciate how going vegan will have a positive impact on your life.

Your other senses become more aware, as well. A vegan friend of mine had to quit her job at a local food co-op after the smell of dairy in the walk-in cooler started to make her sick. Any small spill or open container repulsed her to the extent that she had to resign. It is the same situation when vegans struggle to work in most other food service jobs. Supporting and selling meat, dairy, and eggs when you oppose the consumption of all three is not an easy way to make a living, and most vegans move on to find other work.

All of your senses become heightened—and the most heightened sense of all after becoming vegan is your sense of pride.

It's pretty amazing to wake up every morning knowing that every decision I make is to cause as little harm as possible. It's a pretty fantastic way to live.
—Colleen Patrick-Goudreau

Having cravings for fast food? Want to order something on-the-road? Already missing Taco Bell? Well, you're in luck. Below is an easy-to-use guide on how to order vegan at some of the top fast food restaurants in the United States. Keep in mind that menu options change and that this list doesn't take into account cross contamination, shared oil, or well-trained employees.

1. **Arby's**

   "Chopped side salad with potato cakes, please. Because there is nothing else I can eat here, but I'm dying for your curly fries." Not surprisingly, Arby's isn't a vegan fast food mecca. In fact, like McDonald's (see below), this should probably be considered your last resort.

2. **Auntie Anne's Pretzels**
Little know vegan fast food fact. Auntie Anne's Original, Cinnamon Sugar, Sweet Almond, Garlic, Jalapeno, and Raisin pretzels can be veganized simply by ordering them specially made without the butter. Takes an extra five minutes, but it's worth it for a hot, soft pretzel on the go.

3. **Burger King**
I hope you like fries because that's the only thing that's vegan at Burger King (their limited location veggie burger contains both eggs and dairy). Order up! "Large french fries, please, and hold everything else on your menu." There may be vegetables, toppings, and drinks you can also order, but otherwise, for now, Burger King isn't the greatest option for the traveling vegan.

4. **Carl's Jr. (and Hardee's)**
More brown food! "One order of the french fries, CrissCut fries, hash rounds, and hash-brown nuggets, please." All vegan. In the restaurant, there's an all-you-can-eat salad bar with a variety of vegetables and a three-bean salad. Surprisingly, you can also get the grits (which usually contains dairy).

5. **Chick-fil-A**
Unless you want one of their salads minus the chicken, the only cooked vegan options at Chick-fil-A are the Hash Browns (served only at breakfast) and the Waffle Potato Fries. They do serve a fresh Fruit Cup and Cinnamon Applesauce on the kid's menu, but you have to show ID proving you are ten.

6. **Chipotle**
The Burritos, Bowls, Tacos, and Salads at Chipotle Mexican Grill can be made vegan by ordering sofritas instead of meat.

The tortillas, fajita vegetables, rice, beans, salsas, chips, and guacamole are all vegan, and they are also rolling out a braised tofu that's vegan. Note: their chipotle-honey vinaigrette is not vegan.

7. **Denny's**

   You may not think of Denny's when you think of vegan food, but Denny's serves Amy's brand burgers as the veggie patty for their vegetarian/vegan Build Your Own Burger. The sesame seed and whole wheat buns are vegan, and you can even have fries on the side. This may be your best option if your local Denny's has the burger on their menu and you're craving retro diner food.

8. **Domino's**

   Domino's Pizza offers one vegan crust on their menu, the Thin Crust (the Gluten-Free crust contains honey). Top it with their Original Pizza Sauce and a bunch of veggies. You can order a Garden Salad (hold the cheese) with balsamic or Italian dressing, and you've got a vegan meal in under thirty minutes.

9. **Dunkin' Donuts**

   Most of the bagels at DD are vegan. Order a toasted cinnamon raisin, cinnamon raisin bagel twist, everything, garlic, onion, plain, poppy seed, salt, or sesame, and top it with hash browns, an English muffin, a French roll, or a pretzel twist. Wash it all down with coffee cooled off with almond milk. Not much for nutritional variety, but there are plenty of vegan options to start your day off.

10. **Five Guy's Burgers and Fries**

    Say: "Large fries, please." Five Guy's hand-cut fries are served in an oil-soaked paper bag and will satisfy any salty craving. Keep in mind, however, that out of all the items on their menu (including their milkshakes), the large fries have more calories than anything else they serve. That is, 1,200 whopping calories in a single order. They do offer a veggie sandwich (all their vegetables on a bun), but their bun contains dairy and eggs, so it's not vegan.

11. In-N-Out Burger

In-N-Out Burger may make the best fast food fries on the planet, and there is actually another vegan item that you're going to love. Just walk in and say, "One sandwich, no patty, no spread, and no cheese. Add the grilled onions, please." You'll get one of their secret menu items called "a veggie." The sandwich comes with lettuce, tomato, and onion on a fresh vegan bun and costs around $1.50. Trust me. Order this with their amazing fries, and you're not going to miss the meat.

12. Jack in the Box

"One order of black beans, potato wedges, seasoned curly fries, and breakfast blueberry muffin oatmeal. And a drink cup big enough to put it all in." The list of vegan options at Jack in the Box is so limited, it's hard to imagine making a meal out of it, but they still get high marks for vegan curly fries (I'm looking at you, Arby's!).

13. Jimmy John's

Maybe, as a last resort, you can head to Jimmy John's for a "vegetarian unwich" without cheese or mayo. Basically, it's a veggie sub without the sub (their rolls aren't vegan). Add avocado spread for more flavor and top with oil and vinegar or Italian vinaigrette. All this and a bag of chips.

14. KFC

Surprise! More fries! Order "One order of fries, side of green beans, corn on the cob without butter, and the KFC House Salad with the Golden Italian Light Dressing." It almost looks like a meal if you arrange everything in a strategic fashion before Instagramming it.

15. McDonald's

Lo and behold, the buns at McDonald's *are* actually vegan. Meanwhile, the fries aren't (as I've mentioned earlier, they contain beef). So, on the go, you can get a Big Mac bun loaded with lettuce, tomato, onion, and pickles, and just pretend that "after billions served" they finally ran out of beef patties. Not much else at McD's is vegan (unless your location still serves salads). Keep in mind, the bun contains enriched flour (which contains bleached wheat flour, malted barley flour, niacin, reduced iron, thiamin mononitrate, riboflavin, and folic acid), water, high fructose corn syrup and/or sugar, yeast, soybean oil and/or canola oil. It contains 2 percent or less of salt, wheat gluten, calcium sulfate, calcium carbonate, ammonium sulfate, ammonium chloride, dough conditioners (may contain one or more of sodium stearoyl lactylate, datem, ascorbic acid, azodicarbonamide, mono and diglycerides, ethoxylated monoglycerides, monocalcium phosphate, enzymes, guar gum, and calcium peroxide), sorbic acid (preservative), calcium propionate and/or sodium propionate (preservatives), and soy lecithin. Some of these bun ingredients actually have side effects, so you may want to avoid McDonald's if at all possible.

16. Moe's Southwest Grill

Not unlike many Mexican fast food restaurants, Moe's offers a wide array of vegan options that include organic tofu, beans, tortillas, and rice. Order an Art Vandalay burrito without cheese, a Unanimous Decision taco without cheese, or the Instant Friend quesadilla or the ruprict nachos without cheese—and be sure to add the guacamole. Moe's also offers countless toppings and sides that are all vegan.

17. Panera

Panera Bread's Vegetarian Black Bean Soup is vegan. It has black beans cooked in a spicy vegetarian broth with onions, peppers, garlic, and cumin. Other vegetarian soups have dairy or honey, so be sure to check the ingredients. Have your soup with some ciabatta bread on the side.

18. Papa John's Pizza

At this point on this list, you're getting very hungry. Pick up your phone and call Papa John's right now. I'll wait. Not so much for the thin crust pizza you're going to order with no cheese and tons of veggies, but rather for the garlic dipping sauce, which is vegan. Remember to ask for extra. Like four extra cups.

19. Pizza Hut

I used to *love* going to Pizza Hut, so it's nice to know I can still order the Thin 'N Crispy or Hand-Tossed crust with the regular or sweet pizza sauce and "drag it through the garden." You'll be amazed at how satisfying a cheeseless pizza can be when it's loaded with vegetables. Turns out, the dessert crust at Pizza Hut is also vegan, so just navigate the vegan toppings to finish off your meal.

20. Quiznos

Quiznos has a veggie sub you'll love. Order it "filled with guacamole, black olives, lettuce, tomatoes, red onions, and mushrooms and no cheese." Ask for balsamic vinaigrette instead of red-wine vinaigrette. The vegan bread options include white or wheat, and there's also an herb wrap. Grab a side garden salad and some potato chips, and you'll forget you're vegan real fast.

21. Red Robin

While I've never been to a Red Robin, it offers a Gardenburger that's made with the BOCA Original Vegan Burger patty and can be topped with tomatoes, pickles, lettuce, and Dijon sauce. As if that's not enough to lure me, they also offer vegan Bottomless fries (to add to the size of my bottom).

22. Sonic

"French fries, tots, sweet potato tots, and a side order of onion rings." Sonic. Home of the Vegan Brown Food. It's all these fried potato and breaded dippables that remind me to always pack a to-go pack of Just Mayo. Just because.

23. Starbucks

The menu at Starbucks changes all the time. They've begun offering a variety of nondairy creamers for their coffee bar and specialty drinks. Keep in mind that many of the sugary flavors they use for their extra-fancy drinks aren't vegan. Your best bet at Starbucks is to ask someone what vegan options they have that day and to keep an eye on your barista to make sure she doesn't reach for the whole milk or whipped cream.

24. Subway

Subway is always a savior for me when it comes to finding a vegan sandwich. The Veggie Delite has lots of veggies that you can choose, such as lettuce, tomatoes, green peppers, cucumbers, onions, and even guacamole (for that dreaded upcharge). Have it on their Italian, Hearty Italian, or Sourdough Bread. Top it with oil, vinegar, mustard, deli mustard, sweet onion sauce, or fat-free Italian dressing. If you're not up for a sandwich, order The Veggie Delite Salad and toss in a bag of chips or apple slices.

25. TCBY

Craving froyo? TCBY has you covered. They partnered with the soy milk brand Silk in 2013 to add dairy-free varieties to their menu, and many of their toppings are vegan. My personal weakness? Vanilla Silk frozen yogurt topped with peanuts and peanut butter sauce.

26. Taco Bell

Say, "Bean burrito and Chalupa *fresco* style and sub the beans for meat!" Fresco means no dairy, and they'll put pico de gallo on it. By saying "fresco," you can pretty much eat the whole menu (except the Doritos taco), though it might not hurt to also mention "no cheese or sour cream with vegan rice." Recommendations: bean burrito fresco, tostada fresco (already meatless), Mexican pizza. Add guacamole, since vegans add guacamole whenever it's available in spite of the upcharge.

27. Wendy's

If you go to Wendy's, you can order a Plain Baked Potato and a Garden Side Salad (the dinner salads have chicken and cheese). The salad has mixed greens, grape tomatoes, cucumbers, and bell peppers. Top it with Italian Vinaigrette Dressing but skip the croutons—they have dairy in them, of course.

28. White Castle

Harold and Kumar approve of White Castle's vegan sliders (Dr. Praeger's brand). Order these bite-sized beauties plain or with a sweet Thai sauce.

Another very helpful source for eating out as a vegan is HappyCow.net, an online directory of everything vegan (they also have an excellent app that is always updated).

After reading this chapter, you may suddenly be reminded that this book wasn't written exactly to help you lose weight (though you will), get in shape (though your waistline is going to shrink), or lower your cholesterol levels (though this will happen by default). It was written to help you become vegan. While any of these options could be dismissed as junk food that is clearly not healthy for you, all of them are vegan and will help you transition into your new lifestyle, and new skinny jeans, with ease.

Don't overdo it. Have fun with it. And don't wear skinny jeans (unless you have great legs).

Prove to yourself and your friends that eating vegan is just as exciting and delicious as eating meat, dairy, and eggs and occasionally splurge on any number of incredible vegan ice cream flavors for dessert.

You're going to find that giving up all the foods you thought you loved is a lot easier than you think. In spite of cheese.

Seize the moment. Remember all those women on the Titanic *who waved off the dessert cart.*
—*Erma Bombeck*

Vegans host potlucks. This is a fact of nature. If you're *not* hosting, you're being invited to one. Vegan potlucks are the food orgy of the vegan world.

You can eat everything without having to ask if it's vegan. With one caveat. You've been warned. By hosting or attending a vegan potluck, you're also going to have to abide by a few other rules (knowing the audience, as I do). There is a 100 percent chance you're going to be asked to list your ingredients. Not that they don't believe that the dish is vegan; they just all insist on knowing what they are eating. You may as well write them down on a card to display with your massaged kale salad, even if it only contains kale and the sweat that came off of your fingers while you massaged it. They're going to ask.

And ask again.

I recall my marina days when everyone would bring a casserole of some sort, and the grill would be fired up to cook the meat. Not once, in this setting, did anyone ask for a list of ingredients. You just ate what was brought.

In the world of vegan potlucks, there will also be someone in the group who will request gluten-free options. And nut-free options. And soy-free, oil-free, salt-free, and nightshade-free options. Nightshades are foods like peppers, tomatoes, and potatoes. If you've ever been challenged in the kitchen before, attending a vegan potluck is about to make it that much more interesting.

Our first potluck included ten or so local vegan friends. I made a vegan pizza and a vegan version of a Brazilian cheese bread. It was then when I realized that vegans, as opposed to the whole-food, plant-based population, are *not* in it for health. You can try this out at a vegan potluck at your own risk. You may want to stand back.

Make a big kale salad and put it next to a loaded vegan pizza—and see which is gone first. Or, make quinoa and put it next to a bowl of Tater Tots. Try making a crispy, green salad and put it next to vegan bacon cheeseburger sliders . . . you get the idea. Vegans *love* eating and they love trying new things that, perhaps, they're not customarily making for themselves at home or might consider "taboo."

Since becoming vegan and finding our vegan network of friends, we have hosted a potluck or dish-to-pass a dozen or more times, including Thanksgiving, and have been invited to as many at other locations. The food is always fantastic, and it's truly refreshing hanging out with people with the same interests and dietary requirements as you.

Until an omnivore shows up.

Like a wolf dressed in sheep's clothing, they sneak in. Attached to a vegan they know. Lurking in the shadows. Watching your every move. Ready to call you out.

"What's this?" one such animal eater asked, holding up a fork of barbecue jackfruit. Unripe jackfruit from a can is available in most Asian markets and, when torn into shreds, seasoned, and drenched in barbecue sauce, looks and tastes like pulled pork. (But no one had to die for it.)

"It's jackfruit. Try it. Put in on a roll with coleslaw. Tastes like pulled pork, but no pigs were harmed in the making of it." I'm always trying to make veganism more approachable and understandable to someone who I know is about to strike—by reminding them that they support animal agriculture. I always throw in the fact that they can truly enjoy food without harming another being in the process. This is where vegans and omnivores always collide. The fact that an omnivore could enjoy a fully vegan meal, for some reason, inspires them to mention it would be better with meat. They want to be as unvegan as possible when this argument is used.

This particular omnivore was spring-loaded. She was a cobra, ready to strike at any moment. And she had come prepared.

"Where did you buy this jackfruit?" she asked. Careful now, this question is the string attached to the stick that's keeping the box from falling on top of you.

"At Win-Lee. The Asian market on Route 13," I answered. Short silence. Maybe this was over?

"Vegans," she went on with a chuckle, shaking her head. This was what she's been waiting for. "That's what you vegans don't understand. You're always going on about environmental impact of the meat and dairy industry, and you're always tearing down meat eaters for their choices. Do you have any idea what the carbon footprint of growing, canning, and shipping that single can of jackfruit from China to New York is? Do you?"

My face grew long.

"I didn't think so. Give me locally sourced, humanely slaughtered, grass-fed pigs for my pulled pork any day."

Should I have thrown a match onto the ember and let her know that the canning and shipping in fact do much less environmental damage than any local meat?

I didn't. Which is why I always leave these conversations angry. Angry that they don't hear what they are saying. Angry that they consider eating an animal somehow better than eating a fruit or vegetable. Angry that my compassion is enough to make them angry.

I leave an angry vegan.

In the old days, it was not called the Holiday Season; the Christians called it 'Christmas' and went to church; the Jews called it 'Hanukkah' and went to synagogue; the atheists went to parties and drank. People passing each other on the street would say 'Merry Christmas!' or 'Happy Hanukkah!' or (to the atheists) 'Look out for the wall!'
—Dave Barry

As if getting together with the family during the holidays weren't stressful enough, you're now planning to show up with Tofurky and insisting that all the food is vegan. This probably isn't going to go over well. Meh, holidays are overrated anyway.

The acceptance by family members will vary from family to family. Some are more understanding and sympathetic than others. Take my mom, please. She will insist on a ham at Christmas and a turkey at Thanksgiving even if it means we don't show up. So, we don't.

Year after year we have the conversation, and year after year she insists on serving meat. It's part of her culture and tradition and not something she is willing to part with, even if it means not seeing her son and grandchildren. It's her choice, to choose a dead animal over family. On the other hand, Jen's parents embrace our vegan diets and lifestyle choices, make accommodations, and truly enjoy what we bring to the dinner table. Each Christmas we've spent at their house has been an abundance of vegan goodness, and not once has anyone ever asked for meat to be served.

Since Jen's parents live two thousand miles away and we can't visit during every major holiday, we started our own cruelty-free Thanksgiving tradition, which has grown into as many as thirty vegan outcasts who, like us, may not want to celebrate a traditional Thanksgiving holiday with their own omnivore families.

Thanksgiving is a great time to explore what the holiday means to the unfortunate centerpiece of the traditional omnivore's table: the American turkey. Of course, the other unfortunate aspect of American Thanksgiving, which isn't even given centerpiece status, is the Native American genocide. Turkeys were probably introduced to distract us from this fact. And gravy. Gravy is the great distractor.

Turns out, turkeys are actually intelligent, social, and beautiful wild animals that, at one point in United States history, were on the brink of extinction. Today, wild turkeys still roam forests around the country and can live long, peaceful lives. Domesticated turkeys who are rescued can do so, too—in farm sanctuaries.

Vegans have renamed this holiday "Thanksliving."

Want more interesting turkey facts you can share around your next turkey-free table to convince your own family that a cruelty-free holiday is the way to go? Did you know that, in the wild, turkeys can live up to ten years (as opposed to less than a year on a turkey farm)? These social, playful birds enjoy the company of others and are so athletic they can actually climb trees. The wild ones can, anyway. The domesticated ones climb trees only when they're young because they have been bred to grow so large that, after a few months of fattening up, they're too big to get off the ground. All turkeys relish having their feathers stroked and like to chirp, cluck, and gobble along to their favorite tunes—just like a pet. Would you eat your pet?

There will be forty-five million turkeys unnecessarily killed each November in observance of Thanksgiving and an estimated three hundred million turkeys unnecessarily killed each year for food. As you think about being grateful during the holidays, imagine how grateful three hundred million turkeys would be if they were spared.

Our traditional Thanksliving is now comprised of as many as twenty vegans (and a couple of undercover omnivores). Unless you were specifically looking for it, you wouldn't notice the absence of anything. As soon as the foil is taken off the food, the kids swoop in like hungry little vultures and start to devour everything. Usually, I find myself so trampled by hungry little vegans I can't grab my camera quickly enough to take pictures, so I just stand back and watch as all these dishes evaporate (I always make sure to get a photo of me and my mashed potatoes, though.). I think this is a sign of just how great vegan food is (and, based on their reaction, how raising kids vegan is more than viable).

Our Thanksliving spread covers multiple tables. Each person brings a dish-to-pass, and we pack three six-foot tables to the edges with entrées like homemade Celebration Roast that is stuffed with cornbread stuffing, the perfect centerpiece to the table. Next to the roast are my glorious mashed potatoes, obviously the most popular dish (in spite of the fact it breaks the "no nightshades" rule), as well as Chipotle scalloped sweet potatoes, cranberries, penne Alfredo, and roasted brussels sprouts. I love brussels sprouts. They are like tiny cabbages. Whenever I eat them, I feel like a giant.

Once, we had a traditional Jewish dish, noodle kugel, veganized— the perfect addition to that year's Thanksgiving/Hanukkah mashup. We served kale and quinoa salads and the highlight of the event, four quarts of hot gravy.

Four quarts only, because that's the capacity of my crock pot. Need to get a bigger crock pot. Like Erma Bombeck, I come from a family where gravy is considered a beverage.

What's amazing about nonanimal gravy is that it doesn't harden into a disgusting lump of fat the following day. It stays smooth and edible. Add to this the fact that leftover gravy blended with rice makes the most amazing Thanksgiving-themed risotto. Or, heat it up in a bowl and you've got a creamy, delicious soup. Get on it (the recipe is on page 220).

This meal is finished off with apple and butternut squash pies and homemade coffee ice "cream" for dessert. Everyone goes immediately into a food coma, and since no animals or animal secretions were involved in any of the recipes, the coma feels that much better. As it turns out, the holidays are as tasty as ever, and now we can invite our turkey friends to sit alongside us at the table. Although they have terrible manners.

But Thanksgiving isn't the only holiday to consider. There is Passover, and Easter, and Super Bowl Sunday. Each of these can be veganized with a little effort (and some of the recipes can be found in the back of this book, beginning on page 218). And, of course, there's Christmas. To ring in the festivities at our home, we have written our own Christmas carol, "The Twelve Days of Vegan Christmas." Grab a cup of vegan egg nog and gather round the yule log.

The Twelve Days of Vegan Christmas

On the first day of Christmas my true love sent to me:
A day at Farm Sanctuary.

On the second day of Christmas my true love sent to me:
Two gentle hugs and a day at Farm Sanctuary.

On the third day of Christmas my true love sent to me:
Three french fries (they are vegan, after all), two gentle hugs, and a day at Farm Sanctuary.

On the fourth day of Christmas my true love sent to me:
Four almond milks, three french fries, two gentle hugs, and a day at Farm Sanctuary.

On the fifth day of Christmas my true love sent to me:
Five cheesy Tings (from Pirate's Booty . . . these snacks are dangerous!), four almond milks, three french fries, two gentle hugs, and a day at Farm Sanctuary.

On the sixth day of Christmas my true love sent to me:
Six potlucks buffeting, five cheesy Tings, four almond milks, three french fries, two gentle hugs, and a day at Farm Sanctuary.

On the seventh day of Christmas my true love sent to me:
Seven pants size slimming, six potlucks buffeting, five cheesy Tings, four almond milks, three french fries, two gentle hugs, and a day at Farm Sanctuary.

On the eighth day of Christmas my true love sent to me:
Ate enough protein, seven pants size slimming, six potlucks buffeting, five cheesy Tings, four almond milks, three french fries, two gentle hugs, and a day at Farm Sanctuary.

On the ninth day of Christmas my true love sent to me:
Nine ladies dancing (this one can stay), ate enough protein, seven pants size slimming, six potlucks buffeting, five cheesy Tings, four almond milks, three french fries, two gentle hugs, and a day at Farm Sanctuary.

On the tenth day of Christmas my true love sent to me:
Ten cows a leaping (you *have* to see the video, "Cows Skipping Out to Grass for the First Time" of these British cows leaping around after being let out of their barn), nine ladies dancing, ate enough protein, seven pants size slimming, six potlucks buffeting, five cheesy Tings, four almond milks, three french fries, two gentle hugs, and a day at Farm Sanctuary.

On the eleventh day of Christmas my true love sent to me:
Eleven omnis (omnivores) griping, ten cows a leaping, nine ladies dancing, ate enough protein, seven pants size slimming, six potlucks buffeting, five cheesy Tings, four almond milks, three french fries, two gentle hugs, and a day at Farm Sanctuary.

On the twelfth day of Christmas my true love sent to me:
B-12 supplements coming, eleven omnis griping, ten cows a leaping, nine ladies dancing, ate enough protein, seven pants size slimming, six potlucks buffeting, five cheesy Tings, four almond milks, three french fries, two gentle hugs, and a day at Farm Sanctuary!

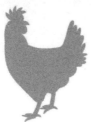

22

THE ANGRY VEGANS

Anger is an acid that can do more harm to the vessel in which it is
stored than to anything on which it is poured.
—*Mark Twain*

Every so often (as you have seen), vegans leave their ahimsa at the door. They go off-script and lash out. Become confrontational (or more confrontational). They grind their teeth, and their blood boils over a conflict or argument involving the vegan lifestyle.

Because they must make peace with the fact that, as children, their parents took them to the local petting zoos to see the piglets and then served pork chops for dinner later that night.

Maybe it's the lack of Omega-3 in their diets or, maybe deep down inside, they are uncontrollably resentful individuals just waiting for a conflict (perhaps their lashing out seems more intense because they are vegan and you don't see it coming). Some of these vegans are professional protesters who disrupt dinners with protest signs and chants of animal cruelty at popular restaurants, cafés, and grocers. Some of these vegans are self-righteous, lecturing, soap-boxing, holier-than-thou activists who will stop at nothing to make their point. Some of these vegans are just fed up and have had enough of defending themselves.

I'm talking about the Angry Vegan. The Angry Vegans who have sent death threats to their favorite vegan restaurant after finding out the very same restaurant was "humanely" raising and slaughtering animals for meat. Early in 2016, forty-year vegan owners of Cafe Gratitude and Gracias Madre in San Francisco were ostracized by vegans after it was discovered that they were raising and slaughtering their own livestock. The café, and others under the same ownership, had an immense, and passionate, vegan following. Once word got out, they were boycotted and held to the flames. By Angry Vegans.

The Angry Vegans who post negative comments on a social media page for a small rabbit farm since they feel rabbits need more standing-up-for-themselves than pigs and cows. Maybe they do so especially because rabbits are fluffy and adorable? These same Angry Vegans will launch an attack against any "sustainable" source of meat and rally the troops to post hundreds of negative reviews and attempt to shut these businesses down.

The Angry Vegans who get enraged when they see an Instagram photo of their favorite "vegan" celebrity eating seafood or promoting a cosmetic line that is tested on animals.

The Angry Vegans who attack a butcher shop when they offered purple sausage as a tribute to the late singer Prince. Since Prince was himself once vegan, these Angry Vegans were twice as upset and demanded the butcher shop offer the same purple sausage with all vegan ingredients.

Then there were the angry vegans who stormed the dentist office and tore down the practice of notorious big-game hunter Walter Palmer, who killed Cecil the lion, a thirteen-year-old Southwest African male who lived in the Hwage National Park in Zimbabwe. Cecil was wounded with an arrow and then killed with a rifle forty hours later. Palmer himself claims that Cecil was killed with a bow and arrow in much less than forty hours after the lion was first wounded. Although Palmer had a permit and was not charged with any crime, the killing resulted in international media attention and caused outrage among animal rights activists and vegans. Angry vegans rallied together to make the doctor's life a living hell, and his practice was targeted online and onsite with protests.

Or consider the life led by Harambe, the gorilla at the Cincinnati Zoo who may or may not have harmed the four-year-old who fell into his enclosure. The zoo was left with no choice but to kill the seventeen-year-old gorilla, and, understandably, everyone got very angry—including many vegans. So angry, in fact, that it brought to light which life was more valuable at that moment in time—the human child, or the teenage ape who shares 93 percent of our human DNA? (By the way, a gorilla belongs in Cincinnati as much as a penguin belongs in Portland. They don't. All zoos should be closed.)

Or the Angry Vegans who splatter red paint on a celebrity's fur coat.

Or the Angry Vegans who picket and protest restaurants serving foie gras.

Or those who call out environmentalists who aren't vegan.

Or the ones who block access roads and parking lots for circuses that are known to abuse their animals.

Or the ones who boycott a TV show because the supposed vegan host launched a shoe line that used leather in their products.

Or undercover Angry Vegans who shed light on inhumane animal treatment at smaller and family-owned or larger factory farms.

These Che Guevara shirt-wearing, sign-yielding, fist-pounding vegans are everywhere, and they are *angry*. All. The. Time. They'll stop at nothing to engage in a toe-to-toe with an omnivore about animal rights and human wrongs. You might say these Angry Vegans give vegans a bad name. Well, they don't. Their actions are justified.

Animals cannot speak.

Imagine if they could. Imagine, for one moment, a Nebraska pig farmer who enters his livestock enclosure, carefully scanning and choosing the one unlucky piglet who will get its throat slit to become that week's bacon and pork. The innocent animal is as terrified of dying as your dog, or as *you* would be. Imagine if, just once, that pig spoke out. In its small, frightened voice, it simply said, "Please, don't."

Two words that could change how we all feel about all animals, forever.

Two words that could potentially turn the world vegan, overnight.

Angry Vegans are speaking up *for the animals*, and while anger and violence are never the answer, the question is what comes into question. These Angry Vegans are standing up for something truly important, and, for this, they have every right to be angry.

23

WHY I STAYED VEGAN: VEGAN BUTCHERS

When you're surrounded by people who share a
passionate commitment around a common purpose, anything is possible.
—Howard Schultz

It was early 2012. So, there I stood, alone at the all-you-can-eat breakfast buffet just two weeks after becoming vegan. I was a thousand miles from home, a thousand miles from The Bet. I needed a cup of coffee and something to eat before heading to the tradeshow floor. No one else was around; it was just me. And this all-you-can-eat football field that consisted of the three most beautiful words ever put together.

Some may argue that the award goes to "peace, love, understanding." Or "I love you." But I beg to differ. Back then, if I had had triplets, I would have named them "Sausage, Biscuits, Gravy."

And, let's be honest here, Gravy would always be my favorite.

I stood at that bar with the ladle *in my hand*, stirring that peppery, light-brown, thick liquid of the gods. Fishing out pieces of sausage and letting them fall back into their warm bath. No one was watching. I could take just one small bite. A ladleful. A plate- or bowlful. Or maybe I would eat it all.

A little angel appeared on my left shoulder. "Don't do it. Think about the animals."

A little devil appeared on my right shoulder. "Go ahead. No one is looking. You've made it for two weeks, you deserve a little bit. Just have a little bit."

"Don't. You'll regret it. You won't be able to live with yourself."

"One bite. Eat some."

I wanted to have a bit; I really did. That savory flavor combo was one of my all-time favorites. The commissary at my old office made it once a week, and they actually named the special after me. I was known to eat four helpings, and after the fourth I always thought I should have one more.

I could justify my actions back then, thinking that I was getting mostly protein from the meat and that my body would use the fuel to burn fat. This may be why I never went to medical school.

I ate none. Not a *single* lick. The devil harrumphed and poofed away, and the angel, who happened to look like Kate Jackson, smiled and flew over to the bar to get me some sliced melon.

Since that moment many years ago, and up until yesterday as I write this, I've been challenged to find foods that appeal to me on that level, especially since my old favorite foods have been reincarnated into their new vegan versions.

One reason I never gave in was that I knew I would be 100 percent committed to this lifestyle from the beginning. I knew that eating a bowl of oatmeal and sliced fruit was *so* much better for my health, and I knew that I wouldn't feel guilty after eating it. I would be guilt-free on so many levels. I was in this for the long haul—and still am. Vegan for life. (The other reason was The Bet.)

Years later, I became part of a bigger community that consisted of like-minded people from all walks of life with the same yearning to make the world a better place. To eliminate unnecessary violence, to heal the planet, and to enjoy a longer and healthier life. This community, for me, extends from Los Angeles to London, and I have made hundreds of friends in cities around the world who are part of this greater good. These are good people who understand me and what I stand for. People to whom I can say, "Thank you for all you do for the animals," without getting a sideways glare.

Our numbers may still be small, an estimated 3 percent worldwide, but we are growing, gaining ground, and making a difference. The number of documentaries focused on plant-based health benefits and the rising popularity of vegan food are appearing all over the world, and *it's not a fad.*

Google's Trends has indicated that more and more people are searching for information related to the term *vegan*. The USDA expects a continued decline in overall meat consumption, with the average American eating 13 percent less meat today than he or she did in 2007. Scientists have found that blood taken from vegans is eight times more effective at killing cancer cells than blood taken from those following a Standard American Diet. More sports venues are adding a wide variety of vegan options. SeaWorld is slowly dying, like the unfortunate marine life they proclaimed they were caring for. People's eyes are finally opening to blatant animal torture, cruelty, and abuse. Private investors are pumping millions of dollars into innovative food startups like Beyond Meat, which had Microsoft's Bill Gates impressed, or Hampton Creek Foods, which garnered the attention of Asia's richest businessman, Li Ka-Shing, along with a $23 million investment. Impossible Foods. Eat Pastry. Fry's Family Foods. VioLife. The list is endless.

You know when Wal-Mart, one of the biggest retailers in the world, expands its organic and vegan food aisle that this is happening. When the stock value of fast food restaurants is on a steady decline. When someone whom you don't expect goes vegan overnight.

And it can happen for you.

Should you go vegan? A) yes; B) A; C) B.

You either approve of violence or you don't, and nothing on earth is more violent or extreme than the meat industry.
—Morrisey

Ever since I went vegan, the number, and quality, of vegan options available at national retailers has expanded a hundredfold. There are entire sections and freezerfuls of vegan meats, cheeses, desserts, and complete meals in the most unexpected places. Whether this is happening as a reaction to a trend or these larger-scale companies are tracking a trend, it's working out great for vegans—and for the animals.

At one point, cheese was the major hurdle for most people who were considering going vegan. Cheese is addictive (and delicious), and the first wave of vegan cheeses was inedible—terrible textures and awful aftertastes led countless vegetarians-turned-vegan back to their cheesy vegetarian ways. This is no longer the case. Vegan cheese companies have popped up in places from California to Greece with a vegan version of every kind of cheese ever created. The taste is outstanding, and more and more companies are setting new standards for other vegan foods.

One of the more interesting recent developments are vegan butchers. These old-school butcher shops sell vegan meats and cheeses, and they look, and operate, like a traditional butcher. Glass cases lined with all varieties of vegan meats that will add flavor, texture, and protein to any number of meaty dishes.

Mock meats, like faux cheese, have come a long way since the first person figured out that vital wheat gluten, which would otherwise be an airless, inedible loaf of bread, takes on all the same flavors as meat from an animal when seasoned and boiled and sliced just right.

When someone tells you that beef, pork, or chicken "tastes great," what they are actually tasting is the right ratio of spices and sauces—all of which are vegan. These flavors are well-suited for developing meat that anyone would take to market.

This little piggy went to market. This little piggy stayed home, this little piggy had roasted beets, and this little piggy had none. And this little piggy went wee, wee, wee, wee, all the way to Minneapolis. Right where my vegan journey began.

Pioneers in the vegan butcher field include Herbivorous Butcher in Minneapolis and YamChops in Toronto. Two vegan-owned vegan butcher shops that got it right from the start.

Walk into the Herbivorous Butcher, and you'll be welcomed with glass deli cases stacked with homemade Italian sausage, piles of pepperoni, mounds of Hawaiian ribs, burgers, and dogs that "teach[es] the world how to love the planet"—all created without slaughtering a single animal. But unlike other meat substitutes that may be frozen or that contain a long list of hard-to-pronounce ingredients, the Minneapolis-based shop's *handmade* products skip the additives.

"We're here to bridge the gap between omnivore and herbivore," cofounder Aubry Walch, with her brother Kale (seriously, that is his actual name), said me to on a phone call right before the airing of the popular Food Network Show *Diners, Drive-Ins, and Dives*. "As much as 70 percent of our customers are omnivores. We've had meat eaters come in and tell us they are buying for their visiting vegan family member, but then they come back a few times a week. Long after the visiting family member has left."

And for the Herbivorous Butchers, it wasn't enough to simply get copious amounts of national attention, from Jon Stewart and Jimmy Fallon to the *New York Times*. The butchers were also contacted by a research scientist at the Minnesota-based Advanced Space and Technology Research Laboratory about helping to create a vegan meal plan for a two-week simulated Mars mission with six astronauts in the Utah desert. If all goes well with the simulation, the astronauts could take Herbivorous Butcher meatless meals into space for real. It's been theorized that alien lifeforms are vegan since they are most likely an advanced being, so these tasty vegan meats will be welcome at the first Thanksliving on Mars.

Oh, and they have hand-delivered vegan goodness to Sir Paul McCartney.

All of the out-of-this-world excitement was happening at Herbivorous Butchers the same week that Guy Fieri from *Diners, Drive-Ins, and Dives* rolled into town in his red Camaro to give their vegan meat a try. Needless to say, it took his tongue to Flavortown.

"He loved it all," Aubry said. "In fact, Guy is mostly vegetarian off-screen, and his sister is vegan." Guy complimented Kale on what they were doing, and I have a feeling that a vegan Food Network show can't be far behind.

On the other side of the border, customers of Toronto-based YamChops run the gamut between vegetarians, "flexitarians," and curious carnivores. YamChops has earned a fanatical following among

Toronto foodies and is carving (ahem) its own niche in the vegan butcher market.

"The idea of doing something with food—plant-based food in particular—has been bouncing around my head for the past eight or nine years," said owner Michael Abramson. "I've been vegetarian for over forty years and vegan for about twelve—and I have also been the primary cook in the house. So, after formalizing my plant-based professional accreditations, we sold our ad agency of twenty-seven years and decided that now, at the age of fifty-nine, was the perfect time to fulfill my plant-based passion.

"I found that there was a big gap in the market in terms of plant-based, center-of-the-plate protein alternatives available. Not wanting to open a restaurant, we opted for a plant-based butcher shop. And the rest, as they say, is history."

In a butcher counter format, YamChops prepares and sells a full range of plant-based protein alternatives, from their popular Szechuan "Beef" and their Ground Beet Burgers to their Sesame-Miso Chick*n, and more.

Additionally, they stock and sell a full range of YamChops packaged products—all delicious—and a range of vegan grocery items including nut-based cheeses, "mayo," and ice cream. They also offer lunch counter service where one can purchase a lunch or light dinner to eat-in or take home.

When I asked Michael if there was any controversy about their shop like what has happened at other vegan establishments trying to "fake" meat, he said, "Ironically, the loudest 'controversy' has been from the ethical vegan community, many of whom are put off by our use of 'meat' words, like *butcher* and *beef*. A small group of vocal meat eaters were also put off by our use of these words, feeling that the meat industry owns them."

I stopped into YamChops during a trip to Toronto for a plant-based nutrition conference, and Michael took the time out of his very busy day fulfilling a catering order for the nearby farm sanctuary by giving me a warm handshake, a bright orange ball cap, and a YamChops T-shirt. It's black. And it's magic.

Times are changing. Michael told me as I was leaving that in the few short years he's been in business, he has already seen a major upswing in the popularity and acceptance of plant-based meats and cheeses.

Not near Minneapolis or Toronto but still want to stock your pantry full of meaty vegan delights? Some of these vegan butcher shops deliver, but you can also check out FakeMeats.com, the vegan version of MeatBucket.com for at-home, online mail order vegan meats. FakeMeats.com started as a collection of their favorite vegan jerky products, and the company grew from there, offering a one-stop shop for a wide assortment of fake meats.

Meanwhile, closer to home, we all love to day-trip to either of the two locations of Strong Hearts Vegan Cafe in Syracuse, New York, or to drive south to visit Eden: A Vegan Cafe in Scranton. Both offer vegan lunches and dinners that satisfy anyone's cravings.

With all these options, why ever eat another animal?

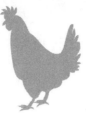

24

A HORSE WITH NO NAME

Be happy with being you. Love your flaws.
Own your quirks. And know that you are just as
perfect as anyone else, exactly as you are.
—Ariana Grande

One of the most difficult parts about going vegan is deciding where to "draw the line." How vegan are you? My advice? Set your dial on Vegan Level 5 as a starting point and, over time, turn it down to three or up to eleven. Set your level to three and you'll likely keep more friends. Set to eleven and you may be living alone with your cats, pigs, and rescue turtles. Over time, you'll find where you're most comfortable. Along your vegan path, you're going to encounter numerous obstacles, challenges, and decisions that predict what level vegan you're really meant to be.

Will you ride a horse?

Will you boycott the horse track?

Will you watch a movie that uses horses in their stunts?

Will you ever watch *Mister Ed* again?

For younger readers, *Mister Ed* was a TV show featuring a talking horse from the late 1950s (also long before I was born, for the record). A sample conversation between Wilbur Post, Mr. Ed's owner, and Mr. Ed would go something like this:

Wilbur Post: [after Mr. Ed makes a great shot in a ring toss game]
Good throw, Ed! I bet you're also good at pitching horseshoes!
Mr. Ed: No, Wilbur, I don't play horseshoes.
Wilbur Post: Really? Why not?
Mr. Ed: Because Mom always taught us kids not to throw our clothes around!

It's funny because (a) horses can't talk; (b) horses don't wear clothes; (c) horses can't throw.

And it's not funny because it actually exploited animals. Mr. Ed was trained like any other animal to do tricks for the camera, and, in his case, nylon string was tied to his mouth and pulled back off-camera to get him to mimic specific facial expressions. It's not as funny when you think about the horse being manipulated this way, is it? As a two-thousand-pound marionette?

I use a horse as an example in this chapter since it's a beast roughly the same size as a cow and since, for some reason, it gets preferential treatment by society. The idea of eating a horse, buying a container of horse milk, or wearing a horsehide jacket is inconceivable to most Americans. But why? It's the same as comparing puppies to pigs: would you eat dog sausage for breakfast? We've been trained over generations and through traditions. Society has our own decision making tied to a nylon string.

Horseback riding and, more so, horse track racing are other examples of how disconnected we often are with our emotions toward animals. Watching Bo Derek ride a horse on the beach in slow motion and watching a horse tumble to its ultimate demise on a racetrack are not as far apart as you'd think. They both require the "breaking" of an animal that otherwise would not welcome a rider on their back.

Horseback riding is *not vegan*.

The most challenging question I've personally posed to vegans, and to myself, is the idea of animals in film. I'm a movie buff; have been for years. Two of my all-time favorite movies are *Butch Cassidy and the Sundance Kid* and *Raiders of the Lost Ark*. Both films, and hundreds more, feature horses being used in a way horses shouldn't be used. While there are standards of practice that "protect" these animals on set, the conditions are still not ideal for the animals, for so many reasons.

From *Ben Hur* to the *Adventures of Milo and Otis*, animals are put in situations that also put them in harm's way. These two films alone are responsible for the deaths of more than twenty animals during filming, but the moviegoer has no idea this happens. As a vegan, are we supposed to boycott these films or look the other way?

To date, the American Humane Association's Los Angeles–based Film & TV Unit is the film and television industry's *only* officially sanctioned animal monitoring program. As a 2013 exposé in the *Hollywood Reporter* revealed, the AHA has often certified a film with the disclaimer "no animals were harmed" even if animals were in fact harmed, so long as they were not *intentionally* harmed. And if a film is produced outside of the United States or without the supervision or approval of this office, it's up to the filmmaker to decide how the animals are treated. I remain undecided on this aspect of veganism. Of course, I want animals to be treated with the utmost care and hope that this is the case, but I still go to movies that feature trained animals. Overall, I think my stance on movies turns my vegan dial down half a notch.

Always let your conscience be your guide.
—Jiminy Cricket

What about some of history's classic cartoon characters? Are any of them vegan? What did they eat on- and off-screen? How did Betty Boop keep her figure?

Let's start with Bugs Bunny. Bugs, of course, lived primarily on carrots and was clearly a herbivore, and it's because of this plant-based diet that Bugs likely had no need to ever visit a doctor. However, he was still strangely interested in occasionally inquiring with them, "What's up?" Perhaps he was wondering what was up with writing all those prescriptions.

Contrary to Dr. Milton Mills's research, it seems prehistoric man was probably *not* herbivorous and may have subscribed to the Paleo Diet, after all. This is shown in nearly every episode of *The Flintstones*, where Wilma and Betty are depicted serving a gigantic bone on the dinner table. This omnivorous lifestyle clearly contributed to Fred's and Barney's obesity, high blood pressure, and overall bad health. Meanwhile, most of the dinosaurs were vegan.

Wile E. Coyote ate birds. It has been documented his diet consisted of only fast food—very fast food. His prey, the Roadrunner, ate desert seeds and plants. It is clear then that Wile E. Coyote's body was probably craving fiber, evidenced by his overall stress level, which is caused by constipation. Mr. Coyote attempted unsuccessfully for years to consume fiber through the Roadrunner and instead got his daily dose of iron from an anvil being dropped from the top of a canyon.

There is a good chance Mickey Mouse and Jerry, of *Tom and Jerry* fame, ate cheese. Instead, Tom and Felix the Cat ate mice. This might explain why these four characters never appeared together in the same film: an R-rating had yet to be introduced. The two ducks Donald and Daffy were omnivores, as was Porky Pig. Luckily, all of these animals were more than free-range, as many of them owned land, cars, and clothing. Except for pants. Ducks don't wear pants.

And what about everyone's favorite sailor on leave? Was Popeye vegan? We all know he had a penchant for spinach. He actually found a way to keep a can, hopefully a BPA-free lined can, tucked inside his Navy uniform for that occasional need for a boost of energy. Like a true vegan, he knew to reach for the leafy greens for that extra punch. Spinach is an excellent source of iron, especially when combined with acidic foods, and it also contains high amounts of lutein and zeaxanthin . . . which, as Popeye shows, provides for strong, healthy seamen.

Ba da bum.

While Popeye may have been vegan, he also had a soft spot for Olive Oyl. And, as we all know, olive oil contains a lot of fat. A lot of any kind of fat, including "healthier" ones, means you're consuming a lot of calories, which leads to excess weight, which in turn leads to increased risks of diabetes, high blood pressure, stroke, many forms of cancer, and, yes, heart disease.

"I yam what I yam and that's all that I yam." Popeye also loved yams. Dr. Greger reports that sweet potatoes are one of the healthiest known vegetables. For me, that settles it: Popeye was a vegan. (But not Popeye's Louisiana Kitchen, although the cajun fries there are. It always comes back to the potato.)

Do the best you can until you know better.
Then when you know better, do better.
—Maya Angelou

How vegan are you?

Will you avoid all food that uses palm oil? The sources of palm oil are rainforests, which are being decimated in numbers that cannot be comprehended. This means palm oil also helps to destroy the habitats of thousands of animals, including our closest relatives: apes. These innocent animals are displaced or killed in the acquisition of this over-used ingredient. The resulting deforestation and loss of natural habitats has threatened critically endangered species such as the orangutan and the Sumatran tiger, and it has increased greenhouse gas emissions. But can you avoid it?

When buying food or cosmetics, it's always good to do your own research, since nonvegan ingredients and processes can appear anywhere. Trust me, you're now going to find palm oil in almost everything. Why? Because even though it is a saturated fat, it is perceived as less unhealthy than the trans-fats it has replaced. Additionally, palm oil is cheap for the same reason that coal is cheap. Of course, the price of the product does not reflect the true cost to others, which is not paid by the producers or the consumers.

Will you avoid white sugar? Most commercially available white sugar is processed using bone char, animal bones that bleach and filter cane sugar. Therefore, most sugar isn't vegan. While countless vegans dip their Oreos in soy milk, they are unknowingly supporting, and consuming, a nonvegan product. Oreos contain sugar *and* palm oil. Despite what I've said previously, Oreos are not technically vegan even though the sum of the ingredients are. If you want to continue eating Oreos, turn down that dial.

Coffee farms, which are only located along the "coffee belt" around the globe and in countries with challenging and unusual terrain, oftenuse mules to deliver the coffee beans up steep slopes that ATVs can't traverse. As many times as you put pressure on your local café to offer almond milk for your cappuccinos and lattes, there's still a very good chance the beans were sourced from a "sustainable farm" that takes advantage of animals, and possibly their people. Knowing this, will you still drink coffee as a vegan? I do. My vegan dial turns down another half notch. It adds up.

Cochineal, from bugs, is used in most food coloring but is not found in kosher products because Jewish dietary laws prohibit the inclusion of insects, or their parts, in food. Shouldn't all laws prohibit this? The latest "trend" is cockroach milk. I'm not even kidding.

Truffles are sometimes dug up by hogs.

Coconuts are sometimes taken down from trees by abused and enslaved monkeys. In Southeast Asia, trained monkeys are capable of harvesting several hundred more coconuts a day than humans. From three hundred to a thousand per day, these monkeys are chained and trained to pick ripe coconuts day in and day out, from the time they were stolen from their mothers, who are typically shot by poachers.

Sharpie markers contain pigments derived from animals. The next time you ask Lindsay Nixon, author of *The Happy Herbivore Cookbook*, to sign your book, be sure to mention this. (Tell her I asked you to.)

Isinglass used in the production of some beer and wine is derived from fish. In fact, many alcoholic beverages aren't vegan. The best source for checking is Barnivore.com, where they've cataloged nearly thirty thousand alcoholic beverages in their massive database.

Heart-healthy omega-3 orange juice contains fish oil and fish gelatin, including tilapia, sardine, and anchovies. Anchovies in orange juice? What will they think of next?

How about some delectable crushed-up bugs in your ruby red grapefruit juice?

Some people claim that the almonds used for almond milk are contributing to the California drought (as compared to the beef and dairy industry in that state, it's not even close) and are therefore not vegan.

Animal-derived sources of Vitamin D3 and L-cysteine exist in nearly every vitamin-fortified food.

Lanolin, from sheep, is used in lotions and shoe polish.

Some margarine contains tallow, the solid fat of sheep and cattle that has been separated from the membranous tissues.

The Prince song "Cream" contains numerous dairy references, even though the artist himself was vegan.

Milk chocolate contains milk. Some dark chocolate also contains milk. Some dark chocolate is vegan but not fair trade or ethically sourced. Cocoa comes from a bean, a bean is a vegetable, and so chocolate is a vegetable. But we vegans care about people, too, and a lot of cocoa is produced on farms employing child labor or even child slaves.

Will you play violent video games that feature killing virtual animals (including human animals)?

Whey as an ingredient in food like bagels, croutons, and breadcrumbs is milk-derived.

Gelatin comes from ground-up bones and horse hooves and is what makes so many candies and jellies so wriggly.

Beeswax and carmine used in makeup are derived from bees and beetles, respectively.

Your condom may be made from sheepskin, and even latex condoms could contain casein, which is derived from dairy milk.

"Natural Vanilla Flavor" in an otherwise vegan ingredient list is sometimes derived from the anal sac of a beaver. Who was the sick scientist who decided to taste beaver junk? And did he have to buy the beaver dinner beforehand? This FDA-approved additive, castoreum, is used in some foods, including many I've been eating over the years. Castoreum is classified by the FDA as "generally recognized as safe" (GRAS). WTF, FDA, GRAS? I am always (trying to be) 100 percent vegan, and now I find out that I have to check ingredients for beaver? Potentially used whenever a vanilla or strawberry flavor is desired. Ew.

And, what about bivalves? Can you eat mussels and clams, since they don't technically have a central nervous system, brain, or parents? Aren't they more closely related to a mushroom? Fine. Eat them. But make sure you're dipping them in vegan butter first—and you're going to have to turn your vegan dial down a full three notches and never mention this to anyone.

Every time you make a choice on whether or not to use or consume products with these ingredients, think about the impact you're having on your own health, the environment, and the animals. If you can eat bread that has honey in it without feeling guilty, then eat that bread. The bread isn't vegan, and you'll have to surrender your vegan identification badge and unlearn the secret handshake. But eat the bread if it's something you really want and if you can live with this choice.

I try every day to make smart lifestyle and diet choices. I avoid all meat, dairy, eggs, and honey in everything I eat, and I will never purchase or wear leather, wool, or silk. I will still watch my favorite movies but would never ride a horse or support any animal racing events or zoos and aquariums. I am confident in my decisions, and I am accountable for my mistakes. I am not perfect, but *I am vegan.*

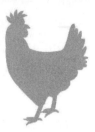

25

BE VEGAN. BE BETTER.

It is amazing how complete is the delusion that beauty is goodness.
—Leo Tolstoy

Vegans have a reputation for being judgmental about everything. Somehow thinking we are better than the 97 percent of the population who aren't vegan. Of course, vegans aren't better than 97 percent of the world but, really . . . we are.

Being vegan simply means you're trying to suck less. In everything you do. You take the time to make decisions that are good for your health, the well-being of animals, and the sustainability of our planet. That *seems* better. Here is a recap:

Being vegan means you're making smart food choices. As you've learned, a large part of veganism is a plant-based diet without meat (or fish), dairy, eggs, or honey. Every meal is planned out and thought through. There is no such thing as stuffing food in your mouth at an all-you-can-eat Chinese Buffet (if someone opens a vegan Chinese Buffet, I will be first in line, by the way). Vegans like myself can get caught in a vegan junk food spiral, but even so, most of these food choices are better for our health and the environment. And much better for the animals.

Being vegan means you truly care for *all* creatures on the planet. We want to end the suffering, torture, and brutal and senseless slaughter of the over 56 million animals killed each year in the United States alone.

Vegans do this by not eating animals and not *supporting* industries that torture and kill animals. As a result, vegans don't wear leather, wool, or silk. *Still sounds better.*

Being vegan means you have more money for fun things, like fabulous vegan vacations. Believe it or not, vegan shopping is far less expensive than shopping as an omnivore. It's said that we "shop around the edges." A plant-based diet leaves you with more money to tuck away.

Being vegan means you are healthier. Some might think we are suffering from a lack of protein and B12, but we really aren't. All scientific evidence has proven that a plant-based diet is better in the fight against all diseases (including cancer and diabetes), obesity, and bad cholesterol levels (vegan diets are 100 percent cholesterol-free). Our arteries are no longer clogged with animal fat.

Being vegan means you look great! Sure, some vegans are skinny and don't look healthy at all. Oh, and some vegans are fat. But we all have great skin, hair, and nails! Also, there is no vegan dress code (aside from not wearing anything that comes from an animal). Wearing old, torn T-shirts with the word VEGAN across the front and vegan sandals with socks are fine. Dressing up professionally in cruelty-free suits or gowns is fine, too.

Being vegan means your appreciation for the little things increases. You have no idea how excited vegans get when they taste a delicious vegan cheese or ice cream. Palates become much more sensitive to different flavors, textures, and combinations. As a result, we really do savor well-prepared food more than most people.

Being vegan means you care. You really do. You care about your own health and well-being, the health and well-being of other humans, the health and well-being of animals, and the health and well-being of planet Earth. This translates to a better world for everyone.

So, if helping to create a better world for everyone doesn't make you a better person . . . what does?

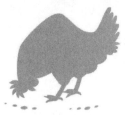

26

PLANET VEGAN

Life can only be understood backwards; but it must be lived forwards.
—Søren Kierkegaard

Welcome to Planet Vegan. The lushest, most peaceful planet in the solar system. A planet where animals live freely among humans without fear of rape, confinement, torture, and slaughter. Planet Vegan, with its crystal clean air, sparkling abundant water, and lavish vegetation from its highest mountains to its wettest rainforests, enjoys a peaceful balance among all life forms.

With its seven million humans no longer bound to unhealthy diets, the planet's ecosystem has stabilized, the once-dwindling polar ice cap has reformed, and all life flourishes for millions of species. Global health crises such as obesity, heart disease, diabetes, osteoporosis, and some types of cancer, which once plagued the planet, have been minimized to a small, and manageable, number of cases per year.

With an entire planet of inhabitants now nourished by only plant-based foods, ten million land animals per year are no longer unjustly caged and farmed for their flesh and secretions, eliminating harmful effects to the atmosphere. Planet Vegan enjoys abundant fresh air and crystal clear water.

And with the elimination of factory farms, Planet Vegan no longer has concerns about animal waste, which in the past caused dangerous levels of phosphorus and nitrogen to leach into the water supply. In such excessive amounts, these deadly levels of nitrogen robbed water of oxygen and destroyed aquatic life in both fresh and saltwater bodies. Parity has been restored, and all life forms enjoy freedom in their natural habitats, from desert to sea.

Humans on this planet, who now enjoy an average life expectancy of ninety-five years of age, wear clothing made from cotton, linen, hemp, and other natural or man-made materials. Personal hygiene products are all organic and have never been tested on animals. All GMOs have been eliminated. Their clean plant-based palates, once dulled from a diet low in flavor-rich fruits and vegetables, have now been reborn. Food pioneers have created delicious dishes designed to spark the appetite of the entire population with ingredients from the earth.

And there's plenty for all. World hunger is a thing of the past. Grain is now readily available to feed the entire population instead of livestock. Droughts are no longer a problem now that animal agriculture has been eliminated.

All zoos and aquariums have been closed and are now the subject of history books, their stories receiving gasps of horror from those who read them. The animals, once caged, now exist in their natural environments and can be observed through sanctuary visits or travel to native lands.

On Planet Vegan, humans practice ahimsa, alongside their other beliefs. A balanced culture that is centered on nonviolence applies to all living beings. Peace has returned to all nations, and those who were formerly ingesting animals are now creating solutions to age-old problems. Violent crime has been eliminated, and prisons have been emptied. It is Utopia.

It took nearly 4.7 billion years for Planet Vegan to fully evolve and for its inhabitants to create the perfect harmony of all its bountiful resources. Evolution works at its own pace.

Planet Vegan is the third planet from the sun. Formerly known as Earth.

You're going to love our restaurants.

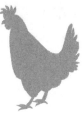

27

THE MEATY VEGAN RECIPES AND THE VEGAN KITCHEN

Vegan food is soul food in its truest form.
Soul food means to feed the soul. And to me, your soul is your intent.
If your intent is pure, you are pure.
—Erykah Badu

When I was an animal eater, I used to love cooking incredible meals for dinner parties, brunches, and cookouts. I was once a guest chef at a Vermont bed and breakfast and who took part in cooking competitions and submitted recipes for other cooks and publications, with some recipes published in *Bon Appétit* magazine. But, alas, those recipes contained animals.

After becoming vegan, I faced the daunting task of converting some of my favorite recipes into their vegan versions. Each of the recipes in this book is specifically designed to help the transitioning vegan by providing something "meaty" and memorable. Again, these may not be the healthiest recipes, but they are much healthier than bacon-wrapped filet mignon with a hollandaise.

And just as delicious.

As a vegan, you're going to be asked over and over why you would ever want to eat something "meaty" when it seems to represent everything you're now against. There are many good answers in varying levels of politeness, but I always tell people that while I miss the taste and texture of meat, I just can no longer enjoy eating it knowing what I know. Truly, with the availability of an endless array of options and replacements, and an ever-expanding selection in restaurants and grocers, there is *no* reason or excuse to ever eat meat, dairy, or eggs again.

As you begin your journey toward a vegan diet, keep in mind that many foods you've eaten your entire life have been vegan this whole time. Start there when planning your meals. Don't think of this new diet as "These are the things I cannot eat anymore," sad face emoji. Think of it as "These are my favorite foods that are already vegan, and the ones that aren't vegan have delicious vegan alternatives," happy face emoji.

Omnivore friends who are hosting vegans for dinner often ask me what they should make. They are usually stressed out about it, and I try to put their mind at ease. My answer is always the same. What would you make if they *weren't* vegan? Now, make the vegan version of that (unless it happens to already be vegan).

I've come alive in the kitchen through veganism, discovering new and challenging ways to bring out flavors in foods naturally and creating dishes that impress all of my friends, vegan or not. This newfound passion for vegan cooking scored me an audition for the tenth season of The Food Network's *Food Network Star* program. I headed to New York City with a cooler bag full of vegan goodness, my rehearsed pitch, and some mangoes. While I didn't make the final cut for casting (as it turns out, another Ithacan was chosen that same season), it was still affirmation that I am someone who can show the world that vegan cooking can be delicious, exciting, and fun to prepare.

I'm still waiting on a callback for my own show, by the way: *The Meaty Vegan Strikes Again.*

Today, I am not only thriving with amazing food every day, I am cooking up a storm all week long (and even more on the weekends), trying out new recipes and creating foods that rival any omnivore's best day. Not only are these meals tasty and filling, they are also packed with vitamins, minerals, and . . . protein. Most of the meals I make are loaded with more protein than you'd find in a meat-based dish—and more than any person would need for a week.

Throughout these recipes, I may refer to things like *milk*, *mayo*, and *butter*. Rest assured, I mean "vegan" in every instance.

I think it's time for the vegan community to stand up and claim some of these words omnivores currently think they own. Since going vegan, I've been inundated with comments from my meat-loving friends about using words that they, for some reason, think are exclusive to flesh eaters. It's time vegans got these words back.

Meat. Or, *meaty*. This word conjures up images of flesh on a grill or a slab of animal at the butcher; however, the word *meat* also refers to the meat of a mushroom or a coconut, or the meatiness of an eggplant or squash. *Meat* does not belong to meat eaters, and the vegan community wants this word back. Especially the Meaty Vegan (me).

Milk. Milk also comes from a coconut and can be made using nuts (and other seeds or rice). Something nondairy can be milky just as much as something nondairy can be creamy.

Cream. Or, *creamy*. While these words connote an image of dairy cream, pretty much anything with a creamy texture can be considered cream. Therefore, we can put cream in our coffee without being called out. You can make an amazing cream sauce with raw cashews or a supersimple creamy soup with butternut squash or cauliflower.

Cheese. Same as *cream*. Cheese can be made with any number of ingredients, and we vegans don't have to explain ourselves (or prove ourselves) if we're serving macaroni and cheese. Or if we put out a cheese tray or serve up a cheesy alfredo (recipe on page 239). It's all vegan. Interesting side note: Miyoko's Kitchen had to use the words "Cultured Nut Product" on their labels and website because using the word *cheese* was illegal in California on products that *don't* contain dairy.

Butter. If we offer butter on something or list it as an ingredient in a vegan meal, it's vegan; contains no dairy. By now, you should know that butter comes from cows, right? A lot of margarine you grew up with is actually vegan, and there are both amazing vegan butters in grocery stores and numerous homemade vegan butter recipes worth trying. You will not miss butter by going vegan.

Bacon. This is now a *flavor profile* and no longer a cut of piglet. I make my bacon with rice paper (recipe on page 218) or mushrooms, and it tastes like bacon. Kevin Bacon would agree.

One word and/or flavor that we cannot truly reclaim is "chicken." We do have un-chicken, chicken-free products, and chick'n, phrases that let us know what to expect, but, for some reason, the word *chicken* will always refer to both the flavor and the animal. *Turkey* is also turkey. Which brings to mind another question entirely.

Would meat eaters ever go to a steakhouse and order *cow*? Or, two fried eggs with a side of *pig*? Words like *steak* and *tenderloin* and *pork* help omnivores further detach themselves from the actual beast from which these foods are derived.

THE VEGAN KITCHEN BASICS

In addition to popular and easy-to-find staples that have been vegan all along (rice, pasta, spices, most bread, etc.), there are a few ingredients you'll always want on hand before taking on these vegan recipes. Of course, buy organic when you can, and if possible join your local CSA to get the freshest fruits and vegetables possible. In my opinion, the ingredients listed here are a requirement—a rite of passage—for vegan cooking.

Potatoes: You might have guessed these would be at the top of my list. Any kind, any size. Always have them on hand to create a tasty side dish or potato salad, whether baked, mashed, or fried. Potatoes are inexpensive and easy to prepare.

Nutritional yeast (nooch): This magical golden dust adds a nutty, almost cheesy, flavor to many recipes and is used in everything from tofu scramble to macaroni and cheese. It can be purchased online or at nearly every well-stocked grocery. It's also an excellent source of that elusive B-12 you've been hearing all about. (Warning: While most popular brands of nooch are fortified with B-12, sometimes the nooch you buy in bulk is not. Read the label.)

Better than Bouillon (vegan version): Or any other organic vegetable-based bouillon. This is great for sautéing vegetables without oil, rehydrating textured vegetable protein (TVP), or making a supersimple risotto.

Himalayan Sea Salt: Or any sea salt you can find. While most advocates for a whole-food, plant-based diet usually avoid added salt and oil, it's nice to have this and a good pepper mill on hand to bring out the flavors in your cooking. Salt is a flavor enhancer and should always be used sparingly. Unless on french fries.

Smoked paprika: I love this simple spice that I add to almost all of my meaty dishes. Add a dash to any recipe to give it that lumberjack flavor without having to swing an ax. It also adds a red color to some of the faux meat recipes you're about to take on. There are variations on smoked spices you can try, and I recommend any of these over liquid smoke.

Rice: White, brown, long grain, short grain, risotto (Arborio). Rice serves as an excellent foundation, or side, for many vegan meals. The Korean dish bibimbap is a rice bowl covered in chopped up veggies. Add wheat-free tamari (soy sauce) or spicy gojuchang (available vegan) and get creative with this simple one-bowl meal.

Wheat-free tamari: This is the gluten-free version of soy sauce, and I always recommend people become accustomed to buying this instead of regular soy sauce. It tastes the same, and if you find out your partner is gluten-intolerant (like I did), you'll score extra points when you pull this out. You can also use Bragg's Liquid Aminos. A similar product in desperate need of a new name.

Beans: Where do I begin with beans? They are so important and versatile that all I can say is 1) dried beans take longer to make and may not be worth the extra effort; 2) canned beans should be organic and in a PBA-free lined can. Adzuki, black, chickpea, fava, kidney, lentil, navy, pinto, or white. Buy all the beans.

Pasta (preferably gluten-free, for the same reason above): As a side or main dish, you could literally survive off a nice brown rice pasta and a million different sauces (with vegetable toppings). Recipes to follow including a simple Alfredo sauce (page 239) that will make you feel guilty about eating all the pasta, as well as a meat-free Bolognese that uses beans. Buy all the beans.

Nuts: Raw cashews and almonds are great for making creams and dairy-free milks. Peanuts are great (I especially love Snoopy), and a lot of people love adding walnuts to bean burgers to make them meatier. Keep in mind that many people have certain nut allergies, especially when preparing meals for potlucks or other occasions, so it's good to ask first.

Texturized vegetable protein (TVP): Texturized vegetable protein, also known as textured soy protein, soy meat, or soy chunks, is a defatted soy flour product, a by-product of extracting soybean oil. It is often used as a meat replacement or meat extender. It is quick to cook, with a protein content far greater than that which comes from animal meat. There are also variations such as Soy Curls that add incredible taste, texture, and protein to any meal.

Oil and vinegar. Again, avoid oil as much as you can, but if you're going to use it (I do), use extra virgin olive oil, high heat sesame oil, or coconut oil. Vinegars come in an amazingly delicious array of flavors; a simple splash added to any salad does wonders.

Maple syrup or brown rice syrup. Excellent sweeteners that aren't pure sugar (for a sugar substitute, try evaporated cane juice, which is a fancy name for "more natural" sugar).

Lemons and limes. While I don't mention it in most of the recipes in this book, having a fresh lemon or lime on hand to squeeze onto pretty much anything adds a burst of freshness that tastes fantastic (same can be said for many fresh herbs like basil, parsley, or mint).

Sauces. Always have the pantry or fridge filled with your favorite barbecue sauces, marinades, tomato sauces, marinaras, and that important full bottle of Sriracha. There's also an amazing spicy Korean sauce called gochujang that is available vegan and that can be added to most dishes.

Spices. Have as many or as few as you like, but it's always best to have the basics on hand. The recipes included here will cover most of the minimum required spices. By all means, load up your spice rack so when you entertain guests in your kitchen; they will feel compelled to say "nice rack."

THE VEGAN KITCHEN TOOL BOX:

There are certain gadgets, tools, and appliances you should have in your kitchen if you're planning to make the recipes in this book and become a masterful vegan chef. Some are required and some are recommended, and all are ones I use most frequently.

Appliances:

- Vitamix (or any other high-speed blender)
- Immersion blender
- Rice cooker/vegetable steamer
- Slow cooker/Crock-Pot
- Mixer (hand or stand)
- Food processor or mini food chopper

Gadgets and tools:

- Nonstick frying pan
- Heat-rated rubber spatulas (small and large)
- Measuring spoons and cups
- Sharp knife set
- Whisk
- Locking tongs
- Strainer/colander
- Microplane grater
- Potato/vegetable peeler
- Mandolin
- Wooden spoons

THE ALTERNATIVES

Today, there is a delicious vegan version of everything. Some are more successful than others in mimicking the original, and I've pretty much tried every one of them at some point along the way. While this list is a great starting point and many are excellent transitional foods, by the time you're finished reading this book, there will be more. The latest and most innovative new products are launched every year at the weekend-long Natural Products Expo (ExpoWest and ExpoEast). This is the world's largest show of its kind, and if you ever have reason or ability to attend, it's worth it. All the major vegan/plant-based food companies are in attendance, and each attempt to one-up the other for innovative new vegan samples.

Please note: Not all of these listed here are available nationwide or in certain retail outlets, but availability in the past few years has expanded into some very unexpected places. Walmart, Target, Aldi, and even some dollar stores across the country are stocking their shelves with vegan goodies. Also, if you have a food co-op near you, they will often special-order items for you (like the time we had them order us a case of Sol Cuisine breakfast patties after they stopped carrying them).

All of these foods are certified vegan and get the Meaty Vegan stamp of approval:

Meat	Beyond Meat, Gardein, Sol Cuisine, Trader Joe's Soy Chorizo, Boca, Field Roast, Tofurky
Milk	Silk (makes soy, almond, and cashew), Pacific Brand, So Delicious, West Soy
Cheese	Chao, Follow Your Heart, VioLife, Miyoko's Kitchen, Daiya, Kite Hill
Eggs	Follow Your Heart's VeganEgg, The Vegg
Honey (sweeteners)	Bee Free Honee, maple syrup, brown rice syrup, agave nectar
Condiments	Just Mayo, Just Ranch, Just Caesar, Just Thousand Islands, Follow Your Heart Vegenaise, Chipotle Vegenaise, Tofutti sour cream and cream cheese, ketchup, mustard, relish, and countless other condiments

Keep in mind that there are also plant-based alternatives being turned into their meaty counterparts every day. Watermelon steaks, shiitake mushroom bacon, jackfruit pulled pork, and any number of nuts and beans can become the protein on your plate.

> *When I see bacon, I see a pig, I see a little friend,*
> *and that's why I can't eat it. Simple as that.*
> *—Paul McCartney*

RPBLT (RICE PAPER BACON LETTUCE TOMATO)

Early in 2016, online vegans went crazy for a rice paper bacon recipe that originated in Denmark. They called it *Lækon*, but we all called it a divine miracle. Most vegans are aware of shiitake mushroom bacon, which tastes surprisingly like bacon but cooks into tiny bite-sized bits. However, this rice paper bacon looks *and* tastes like crisp strips of bacon. It is the perfect addition to a morning tofu scramble, topping on your veggie burger, or the centerpiece of this RPBLT sandwich. This is a fun and easy recipe that gets bacon back in your life within 15 minutes.

Ingredients:
Rice paper (those round disks used to make spring rolls)
2 tablespoon olive oil
Sliced fresh tomatoes
Crisp Romaine lettuce
Soft white bread
Cracked black pepper
Vegan mayonnaise

Cut the rice paper into bacon-width strips. Take two pieces together and dunk them into warm water. They will immediately become flaccid and workable. Don't leave them in too long, since they will eventually become too flaccid. That's what she said.

Heat up the olive oil in your nonstick pan over medium heat. Immerse the two strips into your sauce mixture until coated, then pull them out and shake off excess. Immediately place them into the hot, oiled pan. Hear that sizzle? That means you're doing it right. Turn each over after two full minutes of cooking and cook for an additional two minutes until crisp but not burned. Transfer each to a paper towel and try not to eat them all before constructing your sandwich.

Place four slices of tomatoes and two leaves of lettuce onto one piece of bread. Lay the bacon down in any pattern and crack some black pepper on top.

Slather another piece of bread with vegan mayo. Top the sandwich, slice diagonally (since you're not a caveman), and enjoy.

NOTE: For crispier bacon, toss the strips into a 400°F oven for another 20 minutes on a cookie sheet. Your house now smells like a diner.

HOLIDAY GLUTEN-FREE VEGAN GRAVY

I have always loved gravy. Loved it when I ate meat, and love it just as much now that I am vegan. Gravy on mashed potatoes. Gravy on french fries. Gravy on open-face chicken-free sandwiches. Gravy on coconut ice cream. You could put gravy on a shoe, and I would eat it (provided the shoe was vegan). There is something about that liquid gold that really tops off every savory dish, and this recipe is as good for you as gravy will ever be.

Ingredients:

1 cup shiitake mushroom (or other favorite mushroom) chopped fine

1 finely chopped white onion

3 cloves garlic, finely chopped

½ cup vegan butter

½ cup unsweetened nondairy milk

¼ cup gluten-free vegan Bob's Red Mill All-Purpose Baking Flour

2 cups vegetable broth (we use Better Than Boullion)

1 teaspoon dried herb; or 1 tablespoon each fresh herb (chopped finely):

Parsley

Sage

Rosemary

Thyme (did you sing these last four ingredients?)

Salt, to taste

Pepper, to taste

In a large pan or pot over medium heat, water sauté the mushrooms and onions until soft (¼ cup of water will probably work and most will evaporate during the process). Add the chopped garlic and cook an additional 3–4 minutes, stirring often (the trick to really good gravy is to always be stirring). Did you know the Bob Marley classic "Stir it Up" is actually a song about gravy?

Melt the vegan butter into the pan and stir in the unsweetened non-dairy milk.

In a jar (this is my mom's trick), shake up the flour with ¾ cup of warm water until fully dissolved (*very* important to put the water in the jar before the flour). Pour the flour mixture slowly into the pot and keep stirring. This is already looking like gravy and smelling like gravy, and we're only just getting started.

Pour in vegetable bouillon and lower the heat to a simmer. Add a teaspoon each of the four spices. Keep stirring until the desired consistency. Add water if too thick, and add more magic flour from Mom's jar if too thin. Salt and pepper to taste.

Transfer into a gravy boat with a ladle, or simply ladle directly into your mouth. For even more gravy, quadruple this recipe.

CHORIZOATS (CHORIZO MADE FROM STEEL-CUT OATS)

Bob's Red Mill held a contest a while back to develop an original recipe using their steel-cut oats, and this was my nonwinning entry. Already a fan of soy chorizo, the Mexican spicy sausage used to liven up enchiladas and burritos, I put into play the same concept for making spicy chorizo out of steel-cut oats. Imagine eating endless amounts of "sausage" that's actually good for you. There is a soy-based version of chorizo on the market, but this is a nice departure from soy, and it only takes 25 minutes to prepare. I smuggle a small jar of this into our mostly non-vegan Mexican restaurant and add it to my tacos.

Ingredients:

1 cup Bob's Red Mill Gluten-free Steel Cut Oats

1 tablespoons vegetable bouillon

1 tablespoon extra virgin olive oil (optional)

1 medium onion, finely chopped

1 medium green pepper, finely chopped

4 garlic cloves, pressed or finely chopped

1 6-ounce can organic tomato paste

3 tablespoons apple cider vinegar

2 tablespoons (or more, depending on preference) favorite hot sauce

2 tablespoons fresh cilantro, chopped

2 tablespoons chili powder

1 tablespoons paprika

1 tablespoons smoked seasoning

1 teaspoon ground black pepper

1 teaspoon ground cinnamon

1 teaspoon cumin

Vegan sour cream (optional, but it is worth every extra calorie. I prefer Tofutti brand)

Vegan cheese (optional, but get your hands on some VioLife or Chao).

Cook Bob's Red Mill Gluten-free Steel Cut Oats according to package (1 cup oats, 3 cups water) in a pot. Add vegetable bouillon just before adding oats, and cover with a lid (it will take 20 minutes to cook covered, stirring occasionally).

Heat olive oil in a skillet (you can do this step oil-free if you're one of those people). Sauté onions, pepper, and garlic until soft. Stir in tomato paste and lower heat. Add apple cider vinegar, hot sauce, cilantro, and stir. Continue stirring over low heat for 5 minutes.

Combine all dry ingredients in separate bowl. Stir into the tomato mixture and set aside.

Once Bob's Red Mill Gluten-free Steel Cut Oats are done (can be left a little chewy), combine it with the tomato mixture in a large bowl. You now have enough Chorizoats to fill six burritos, tacos, or quesadillas. The Chorizoats are also an excellent addition to vegan chili. Or cook further over medium heat in a frying pan and add as a healthy, spicy vegan pizza topping.

PINES BEETS BURGERS

Everyone loves a burger—and a burger loaded with toppings is even better. This vegan bean burger is packed with protein and, when dressed in tomato, lettuce, and vegan Thousand Islands dressing, is as satisfying as any beef burger you've tried. You can make a full batch of these and freeze them for grilling down the line.

Ingredients:

1½ cups cooked brown rice

1 15-ounce can organic lentil beans

1 15-ounce can of organic beets

2 tablespoons milled flaxseed (soak in 6 tablespoons warm water for two minutes)

½ teaspoon chili powder

½ teaspoon smoked paprika

½ teaspoon garlic powder

½ teaspoon onion powder

½ teaspoon salt

¼ cup gluten-free vegan Bob's Red Mill All-purpose Baking Flour

4 tablespoons olive oil, for browning burgers

Add all ingredients into a food processor (except the flour and olive oil) or add them in a large bowl and use an immersion blender (my preference). Blend together without losing too much texture (probably 45–60 seconds).

Cover and refrigerate for about fifteen minutes. Remove from the refrigerator. Shape the mixture into patties using flour on your table and to dust your hands to keep the stickiness to a minimum. This will also form a crispy crust when you fry. You will get about six patties, depending on the size. You might want to line a sheet pan with wax or parchment paper to set these aside as you make them. Dust with extra flour as needed.

Heat a large pan over medium heat with the olive oil. Cook the burgers for about 3–5 minutes on each side, until crisp and heated through. Dress. (The burgers. I hope you weren't making these naked.)

CARROT HOT DOGS

Hot dogs are notoriously bad for you and contain any number of strange body parts. These carrot hot dogs contain one main ingredient: a carrot. Find a big, fat carrot, or four, and "carve" them into the shape of a hot dog with a paring knife (if you want to be really authentic). These carrots take 24 hours to marinate overnight, but once they are ready, they can be fried or easily rolled onto the grill. Once marinated, they take around 20 minutes to cook. Imagine eating these endlessly at your next tailgate party loaded with sliced onions, sauerkraut, spicy mustard, and relish—with zero guilt.

Ingredients:

2 large carrots, peeled, and carved to look like hot dogs
¼ cup wheat-free tamari (soy sauce)
1 tablespoon rice vinegar
1 tablespoon sesame oil
½ tablespoon apple cider vinegar
1 tablespoon smoked paprika
2 cloves garlic, minced
¼ teaspoon black pepper
⅛ teaspoon onion powder
½ teaspoon sea salt
Olive oil, for sautéing
Hot dog buns and toppings

Boil carrots for approximately eight minutes, or until fork tender but not mushy. After removing the carrots from the boiling water, run them under cold water to stop the cooking process. While the carrots are cooking, whisk together the rest of the ingredients (except for olive oil and hot dog buns and toppings).

Combine the carrots and the marinade in a gallon-size zipper bag (use two, putting one in the other, in case they leak). Shake until the carrots are coated with the marinade. Place the carrots on a plate in the refrigerator for at least 24 hours, turning them and admiring them all night long. Now go to bed.

Wake up. It wasn't a dream; your carrots are ready. To cook them, coat a nonstick skillet with olive oil. Turn the heat to medium and place the carrots and about ½ cup of the marinade into the skillet. Heat the carrots for approximately 8–10 minutes, or until they're warm. For added crunch, try frying the finished carrot dogs in a tablespoon of oil to further darken the edges. They are now ready to eat or bring to the outdoor barbecue!

BBQ and Tailgating Tips

Being vegan and hosting or attending barbecues or tailgating parties doesn't mean you have to resort to hummus and chips while others flip burgers and dogs. In addition to countless off-the-shelf veggie burger options, there are many homemade recipes that will satisfy any sun-scorched vegan, and perhaps surprise an omnivore or two. Bring your favorite veggie burgers (p. 224), carrot hot dogs (p. 225), or portobello mushrooms (p. 234) to grill and a bunch of sides, and crack open a (vegan) beer!

Keep in mind that so many BBQ foods are already vegan:

> Watermelon/fruits
> Carrots/celery and pepper trays
> Corn on the cob (bring the vegan butter)
> Hot dog and hamburger rolls
> Relish, sliced onions, sliced tomatoes, lettuce
> Potato chips/tortilla chips
> Salsa and guacamole
> Ketchup, mustard, and hot sauce
> Baked beans

Other BBQ and tailgating favorites that can be easily made vegan are:

> Macaroni salad (use vegan mayo)
> Potato salad (use vegan mayo)
> Coleslaw (use vegan mayo)
> Ranch dip (p. 247)

TOFU SCALLOPS

I felt compelled to include one "seafood" recipe in this book. These simple tofu scallops make an excellent side or starter, are fun to make, and require zero shucking. Hey, why not wrap these in bacon (now that you know how to make vegan bacon)?

Ingredients:

1 block extra-firm tofu, pressed and drained

2 tablespoons wheat-free tamari

2 tablespoons vegetable broth powder (we use Better Than Bouillon)

¼ cup gluten-free vegan Bob's Red Mill All-Purpose Baking Flour

Sea salt

1 sheet (equivalent) sushi nori roll, crumbled into flakes

Old Bay Seasoning

2 tablespoons olive oil

2 tablespoons vegan butter

Lemon slices

White rice

Cut the block of tofu in half, then cut each half in two along the width. You will have four rectangles if you did your math right. Using a shot glass or any other 2- to 3-inch-wide circular kitchen thingy, punch out circles for each scallop. You're going to have some leftover tofu, but you'll be using that in your tofu scramble tomorrow morning, so just stick it in the fridge.

Combine the tamari and the vegetable broth in a shallow bowl to make a marinade. Marinate the tofu pucks in the fridge for at least 30 minutes in a covered container. After 30 minutes, remove from the marinade and shake off excess moisture before lightly coating all sides in flour.

Sprinkle the "scallops" with a bit of salt, nori flakes, and Old Bay Seasoning on both sides.

Heat an oiled large nonstick skillet over medium-high heat. Add butter to the pan and heat until sizzling. Slowly (best with tongs) place each scallop on the pan and let it sear on each side before turning. Fry each for about three minutes on each side, adding butter and more Old Bay for flavor (and to make sure they aren't sticking).

Serve with lemon slices on a bed of white rice.

MEATY VEGAN CHILI

Vegetarian chili is nothing new. What makes this recipe so special is that it's so easy to make. Line up all these ingredients, grab your biggest pot, and build this chili from scratch. Serve with shredded vegan cheese and vegan sour cream on top, and you'll never miss chili con carne again. Prep and cooking time: 30 minutes.

Ingredients:

Olive oil

1 large onion, chopped

2 cloves garlic, chopped

1 each green and red pepper, chopped

1 15-ounce can kidney beans, rinsed and drained

1 15-ounce can black beans, rinsed and drained

1 large can of organic diced tomatoes

3 tablespoons chili powder

3 tablespoons smoked paprika

¼ cup favorite vegan barbecue sauce

1 package premade vegan beefy crumbles (optional, both BeyondMeat and Gardien make excellent products loaded with taste and protein)

One jalapeño pepper, chopped with seeds reserved

Vegan cheese (optional)

Vegan sour cream (optional)

In a large pot, add a gurgle of olive oil. Once hot, add the onions, garlic, and green and red peppers and cook until just tender, about 3 minutes. Pour both cans of rinsed beans into the pot and give it a good stir.

After a couple minutes, add the diced tomatoes, chili powder, smoked paprika, and barbecue sauce. Stir. See? That was easy, right? Add more chili powder, since we are making chili after all. After about 20 minutes on low heat, pour in the bag of crumbles (optional), cover, and cook down for an additional 10 minutes, stirring occasionally.

Chop the jalapeño and add as many seeds into the pot as you like to adjust the heat. Garnish the top of your chili with the chopped jalapeño and any other vegan toppings you desire (sour cream and cheese recommended).

TOFU WINGS

Many restaurants are beginning to offer tofu wings, and the styles and variations are pretty broad. Essentially, pressed tofu is cut into triangles, floured, fried, and finished with Buffalo wing sauce. It will probably take less than 40 minutes from start to finish. Serve with celery sticks and vegan ranch dressing.

Ingredients:

1 14-ounce block of extra-firm tofu (pressed for 15 minutes)
3 tablespoons cornstarch
1 tablespoon garlic powder
1 tablespoon smoked paprika
½ teaspoon sea salt
2 tablespoons olive or vegetable oil
Favorite vegan BBQ or wing sauce

To press the tofu: Remove the tofu from its packaging and squeeze out excess water. Place the block on a towel on a plate, fold the towel over the top, put another plate on top, and cover with those gym weights you don't use any more so the tofu is squashed to almost half its original height. Let it drain for at least 15 minutes. Pat the tofu dry.

Slice the pressed tofu into ½-inch-thick triangles, rectangles, or perfect squares (up to you). You should end up with about 10 pieces total.

Mix cornstarch, garlic powder, smoked paprika, and sea salt into a shallow baking dish. Coat each piece of tofu with the mixture on all sides (add more cornstarch as needed). Lay these out on a baking sheet or any other flat surface while you get a skillet nice and hot with some vegetable oil. Your oil is hot enough when a drop of water dances like Tina Turner.

Add the tofu in a single layer. It should immediately sizzle and sear. Pan-fry each piece of tofu until golden on all sides. Coat in wing or BBQ sauce and eat!

CAULIFLOWER BITES

This is a nice break from all that soy, isn't it? These baked (or fried) beauties are also amazing chicken wing replacers. Sliced cauliflower takes on the shape of Buffalo wings and are prepped in a hot oven (which is also a nice break from all that frying). Turned once, they are ready to plate and drown in BBQ sauce. Total prep and cooking time: 45 minutes.

Ingredients:

¾ cup gluten-free brown rice flour
½ cup unsweetened nondairy milk
2 tablespoons garlic powder
2 tablespoons smoked paprika
Salt, to taste
Pepper, to taste
1 large head of cauliflower, sliced into "chicken wing" shapes
Vegan BBQ sauce (optional)

Preheat oven to 450°F. Whisk together flour, nondairy milk, garlic powder, smoked paprika, salt, and pepper together in a bowl until the batter is smooth and somewhat runny.

Add sliced cauliflower to batter and mix until cauliflower is coated (get your hands in there). Spread onto a parchment paper on a baking sheet (or you can lightly grease the baking sheet).

Bake for 10 minutes, turn each piece over, and bake for another 15 until edges start to become crisp. Pour into bowl and mix with vegan wing or BBQ sauce. Eat with your fingers like your mama told you not to.

SUPER SIMPLE TACO SALAD

I used to make this once a week when I was a carnivore. If you can find a taco bowl to eat this out of, go for it, but it's just as good in a regular bowl. The hot ground "beef" on top of the cold romaine lettuce makes this fun to eat. This recipe will make one large salad enough to share. Add as many or as few jalapeño peppers as you can take.

Ingredients:

1 head Romaine lettuce, finely chopped

¼ cup vegan ranch dressing (recipe on page 247)

1 large tomato, diced

1 small red onion, diced

Oil, for frying

1 bag vegan beef crumbles (BeyondMeat or Gardein brand), defrosted

1 package taco seasoning (most are vegan)

¼ cup barbecue sauce

Avocado, diced

Jalapeño peppers, chopped (remember, it's the seeds that are hot)

Vegan sour cream

Place chopped lettuce into a large bowl and toss with ranch dressing. Toss in diced tomato and red onion and set aside.

In a lightly oiled frying pan, heat beef crumbles and stir in taco seasoning and barbecue sauce. Transfer tossed salad into bowls (it should make two servings) and top with diced avocado and jalapeño peppers. Spoon a full cup of beef onto the lettuce, top with sour cream, and enjoy!

SPICY TACOS (WITH GROUND "BEEF")

Everyone loves tacos. Turn your head and crunch. The great thing about building a taco is that you can add as little or as much of your favorite ingredients to suit your taste. It's also an excellent way to get more greens and veggies into your body. Total prep and cooking time: 40 minutes.

Ingredients:

12 corn tortillas or taco shells

1 teaspoon olive oil

1 onion, chopped

2 tablespoons chopped and seeded jalapeño

1 12-ounce package soy chorizo (or use the Chorizoats recipe on page 222)

1 15-ounce can vegetarian refried beans

Large tomato, diced

Fresh cilantro, chopped

Vegan cheese, shredded

Vegan sour cream

Avocado, diced

Warm your taco shells or corn tortillas in a low oven while making this recipe.

Heat oil in large nonstick skillet over medium heat. Add one half of the sliced onion and all the jalapeño pepper and sauté until tender, about 10 minutes. Add soy chorizo and cook until beginning to brown in spots, stirring often, about 5 minutes.

Meanwhile, cook beans in a small saucepan with the remaining half of the chopped onion over low heat until heated through (15 minutes), stirring occasionally.

Fill your tortilla or taco shells with all this goodness and sprinkle the top with diced tomato and cilantro. Top with cheese, sour cream, and diced avocado.

PORTOBELLO STEAKS

Great on the grill or under the broiler at home. These big fatties take on a steak-like personality and are a welcome addition to an entrée, or squished between two pieces of bread, or served alongside potatoes and onions. Don't have a grill? Preheat your broiler to 500°F and bake mushrooms for 3–5 minutes on each side. Make sure you take the battery out of your smoke detector first. Place mushroom on a plate with some sautéed greens and a baked potato. Splash on some fancy A1 sauce—only if you're fancy. Total prep and cooking time: 1 hour.

Ingredients:

½ cup balsamic vinegar
½ cup olive oil
¼ cup fresh lemon juice
¼ cup chopped fresh parsley
3 garlic cloves, minced
2 tablespoons smoked paprika

6 large, fresh portobello
    mushroom, caps brushed clean
Oil, for the grill
A1 Steak Sauce (optional—and
    vegan)

In a large, shallow bowl, stir together the vinegar, olive oil, lemon juice, parsley, garlic, and smoked paprika. Add the mushrooms and turn to coat. Let stand at room temperature for about 1 hour, turning once. Remove from marinade before grilling/broiling in the oven.

Prepare a charcoal or gas grill for direct grilling over medium-high heat. Oil the grill rack.

Place the mushrooms, flat-side down, over the hottest part of a charcoal fire or directly over the heat elements of a gas grill. Cook, turning once, until moist on the underside and just firm to the touch on the top, 4–6 minutes per side. Arrange the mushrooms on individual plates and serve hot with roasted potatoes and onions.

SPAGHETTI BOLOGNESE

This is admittedly the easiest recipe in the book and a great way to get beans and fiber into your colon. Grab a jar of your favorite pasta sauce (vegan) and some spaghetti (most dried pasta is vegan), stir in a jar of lentil beans, and you have the start of a very convincing, high-protein vegan spaghetti Bolognese.

Ingredients:

1 package spaghetti
Olive oil, for sautéing
¼ cup wheat-free tamari
1 can lentil beans

1 jar of your favorite vegan marinara sauce
Vegan Parmesan cheese (optional)

Boil pasta according to the directions and drain.

In the same pot, add a little olive oil, tamari, and beans. Cook until hot over medium heat, about 3 minutes. Add the marinara sauce and stir. Either mix your cooked spaghetti into the sauce or do it the other way around—just get that sauce mingling with the pasta while they're both still hot!

Top with vegan Parmesan.

CYBIL SHEPHERD'S MUFFIN PIES

Shepherd's pie, a casserole of mashed potatoes that blankets a mound of ground beef, peas, and carrots swimming in gravy, is one of the easiest recipes to make vegan. This recipe takes the classic one step further by transforming it into bite-sized minimuffins of goodness.

Ingredients:

4 large baking potatoes, washed, peeled, and diced

3–4 tablespoon vegan butter

Salt, to taste

Pepper to taste

1 medium onion, diced

2 cloves garlic, minced

1 tablespoon olive oil

1 16-ounce can of lentil beans

2 cups vegetable stock

2 teaspoon fresh thyme, or 1 tsp dried thyme

1 10-ounce bag frozen mixed veggies: peas, carrots, green beans, and corn

¼ cup all-purpose gluten-free flour

Bring a pot of salted water to a low boil, add diced potatoes, and lower to medium high heat. Cover and cook for 20–30 minutes or until they slide off a fork very easily.

Once cooked, drain the potatoes and add back to the pot to evaporate any remaining water, then transfer to a mixing bowl. Use a masher or large fork to mash until smooth but not runny. Add desired amount of vegan butter and season with salt and pepper to taste. Set aside and allow to cool.

Preheat oven to 425°F and grease the inside of an 8-cup cupcake tin. Carefully add potato to each cup, lining the bottom and the edges, and shape a rounded indent (like a little "potato bowl") in each cup to make space for the filling.

In a large saucepan over medium heat, sauté onions and garlic in olive oil until lightly browned and caramelized, about 5 minutes. Add a pinch each of salt and pepper. Add the lentils, vegetable stock, and thyme, and stir. Bring to a low boil, then reduce heat to simmer.

After 10 minutes of cooking, add the frozen veggies and stir. Taste and adjust seasonings as needed. Melt in a tablespoon of vegan butter, and dust the top with flour, adding slowly and stirring constantly to create a thick gravy. Set 1 cup of gravy aside.

Bake at 425°F for 10–15 minutes. Remove from oven to let it cool for 10 minutes. The longer it sits, the more it will thicken and the easier it will be to remove from the cupcake tin. Using a butter knife, release the potato around the outer edges, then remove with a rubber spatula and serve. Top with extra gravy.

MANBURGER HELPER

I went there. My dad used to feed us Hamburger Helper, and I actually ate a lot of it as an adult. It was easy and filling, and it came in a variety of flavors. This recipe is for the Stroganoff variety to pay homage to the Swedish side of my family.

Ingredients:

2 cups unsweetened nondairy milk

1 bag shredded vegan cheddar cheese

½ cup onion, diced

2 cloves garlic, minced

1 cup frozen or fresh spinach, chopped

3 teaspoons vegetable broth

1 15-ounce can Italian diced tomatoes

3 teaspoons Italian seasoning

½ tsp garlic powder

½ tsp salt

10-ounce pasta (fusilli recommended), cooked according to directions

1 bag vegan beef crumbles, defrosted

Prepare cheese sauce by heating nondairy milk over low heat in a large pot and stirring shredded cheddar cheese until fully incorporated. This will make 1½ cups of cheese sauce. Set aside. This same pot will be used to stir all the ingredients together later.

Over medium heat, sauté the onion, garlic, and spinach in vegetable broth until the onion is translucent. Add the diced tomatoes, Italian seasoning, garlic powder, and salt. Simmer on low heat for 15 minutes and transfer to large pot.

Stir in the cooked pasta, beefy crumbles, and cheese sauce and continue heating over medium heat for an additional 10 minutes.

WHITE ALFREDO LASAGNA

This recipe is a fun project—you stack layer upon layer of ingredients, sauces, and vegan cheese to build the ultimate three-layer white Alfredo lasagna.

Ingredients for Alfredo sauce:

1½ cup soaked (for 4 hours) raw cashews, rinsed
6 fresh organic basil leaves
½ cup Follow Your Heart mozzarella shreds
¼ cup nutritional yeast
4 cloves garlic, chopped
1 teaspoon sea salt

Ingredients for filling:

½ tablespoon olive oil
1 cup chopped organic broccoli florets
1 cup chopped red onion
5 cloves garlic, chopped
1 brick organic firm tofu
½ cup nutritional yeast
½ lemon, juiced and zested

Ingredients for lasagna:

2 boxes lasagna noodles (gluten-free)
Sea salt, for boiling
1 tablespoon olive oil, plus more to grease
1½ cups Follow Your Heart mozzarella shreds
Italian seasoning
Fresh organic basil leaves for garnish
Cherry tomatoes, sliced

Making the Alfredo sauce:

Rinse soaked cashews thoroughly and add to Vitamix or any other high-speed blender/food processor. Add 1 cup fresh water to fully cover cashews, then add 6 fresh organic basil leaves, Follow Your Heart mozzarella shreds, nutritional yeast, garlic cloves, and sea salt (add more if desired). Blend until creamy.

Making the filling:

Heat olive oil in a pan. Sauté broccoli, onions, and garlic until tender and set aside. In your Vitamix or high-speed blender, blend the firm tofu, nutritional yeast, and juice and zest of the lemon until consistency matches ricotta cheese. Transfer to large bowl and fold in the broccoli and onion mixture.

Making the lasagna:

Cook gluten-free lasagna noodles in 6 cups boiling salted water (add olive oil to avoid sticking) until just pliable. Rinse with cold water and set aside.

Grease more oil on a 9 x 12 glass lasagna pan and pour in Alfredo sauce to fill the pan ¼ inch high. Add first layer of noodles, pressing lightly into the sauce. Spread on a layer of filling over the noodles and pour another light coating of the Alfredo sauce. Continue building lasagna in this way until you reach the top of the pan. Sprinkle the entire top of the lasagna with Follow Your Heart mozzarella shreds and Italian seasoning. Cover with aluminum foil.

Bake lasagna at 375°F for 45 minutes, covered. Uncover and broil for an additional 10 minutes until it starts to crisp and get bubbly. Let it cool for 10 minutes before cutting into squares. Serve topped with fresh chopped basil and sliced cherry tomatoes.

HULK PESTO

This versatile sauce was created as a way to introduce more vegetables to our kids' dinner. Making a green pesto sauce from kale puts the superfoods right into their pasta or on top of a sandwich. You can also try a broccoli variation.

Ingredients:

1 small bunch kale

¼ cup olive oil for the blender, plus extra to braise kale

1 clove of garlic

1 lemon

¼ cup nutritional yeast

3 tablespoons chopped fresh basil

2 tablespoons pine nuts, plus extra to garnish (optional)

2 tablespoons vegan Parmesan cheese, plus extra to garnish (optional)

Salt, to taste

Pepper, to taste

1 bag of whole wheat or gluten-free penne pasta

Braise the kale in a little olive oil. Add one cup of water and cover over medium heat for five minutes. Transfer kale to ice bath. This will make 2 cups of cooked kale.

Add kale to a high-speed blender with ¼ cup olive oil, one clove garlic, juice of one lemon, nutritional yeast, basil, and ¼ cup water. Blend on high speed for one minute.

Use more water to thin or more nutritional yeast to thicken to desired consistency. Add pine nuts, reserving extra to garnish (optional) and vegan Parmesan, reserving extra to garnish (optional). Blend until done. Salt and pepper to taste.

Transfer pesto sauce into a large pan and fold into gluten-free penne pasta. Pesto also makes an amazing spread on sandwiches. Garnish with extra pine nuts and vegan Parmesan (optional).

VEGAN CORN DOGS

To simplify the process, put the corn dog batter into a tall glass and dip the hot dogs in. The real challenge is deep frying these if you don't have a deep fryer; you can also fry them in an inch of oil in the pan that has been heated to 350°F, turning carefully as you cook.

Ingredients:

Oil, for frying (vegetable recommended)

1 ¼ cup white flour

¾ cup fine cornmeal

1 tablespoon vegan egg replacer or ground flax

4 tablespoon sugar

1 teaspoon baking powder

1 teaspoon salt

1 cup unsweetened nondairy milk

6 corn dog sticks or chopsticks

6 vegan hot dogs

Gluten free flour, for dusting

Heat oil in a fryer to 350°F. Mix all the dry ingredients and add 1 cup of unsweetened nondairy milk. Mix until smooth. Add additional milk if needed until batter has a consistency of pancake batter.

Insert sticks into vegan hot dogs and roll them in flour (this helps the batter to stick). Brush off excess flour. Dip in batter, shake off excess, and gently lower into hot oil. Fry for 3–5 minutes until golden brown. Serve hot with a side of yellow mustard.

SMOKY PULLED POKE JACKFRUIT

One can of unripe jackfruit from a local Asian market sautéed with the right blend of spices and fried, baked, or barbecued will make the perfect pulled "pork" sandwich. Serve on a grilled roll with a dollop of spicy mustard and some homemade coleslaw, or use as a filling in tacos or burritos.

Ingredients:

1 16-ounce can unripe jackfruit (most Asian markets sell this; look for the kind not packed in syrup)

Oil, for sautéing

1 cup chopped onion

1 clove garlic, chopped

1 cup chopped shiitake mushrooms

1 cup diced red and/or orange peppers

1 teaspoon sea salt

1 teaspoon smoked paprika

1 cup vegan barbecue sauce

To garnish (optional):

Raw onion, chopped

Jalapeño, chopped

Lettuce, shredded

Vegan cheese, shredded

2 tablespoons chipotle sauce

Preparing the jackfruit is the hardest part of this recipe. Drain the can and rinse. On a cutting board, cut off the "knuckle" of each, leaving the "meat" just loose enough to come apart in the pan.

Oil a nonstick pan and sauté the chopped onion and garlic until soft. Stir in the mushroom and peppers and cook on medium for 10 minutes. Stir in the sea salt, smoked paprika, barbecue sauce, and the jackfruit.

Continue cooking until the edges of the jackfruit begin to burn. Serve hot in a taco shell with additional chopped raw onion, jalapeños, shredded lettuce, and shredded vegan cheese. You can also bring the jackfruit to a cookout and heat it up again on the coals for a truly authentic flavor.

NANA'S ITALIAN MEATBALLS

I grew up eating and loving meatballs. Being half-Swedish and half-Italian meant I had to choose between two flavors at any given meal. It also meant my friends referred to me as the Swedish Meatball. While I do love Swedish meatballs and the creamy gravy involved, I had to go with the Italian side of my family on this one (otherwise, someone might get whacked). These meatballs taste great in white gravy with vegan sour cream.

Ingredients:

1 tablespoon flaxseed

3 tablespoon warm water

1 12-ounce block tempeh

2 shallots, chopped

2 garlic cloves, chopped

2 tablespoons gluten-free, vegan Worcestershire sauce

2 tablespoons vegan Parmesan or nutritional yeast

2 tablespoons fresh parsley, chopped

1 teaspoon dried oregano

1 teaspoon dried basil

1 teaspoon sea salt

⅓ + ¼ cup gluten-free bread crumbs

1 jar favorite vegan marinara sauce

Vegetable oil, for frying

Mix flaxseed and warm water in a small bowl and let sit for about 10 minutes. This is your binder. Break up the tempeh and add it to a food processor. Add the shallots, garlic, Worcestershire sauce, and Parmesan or nutritional yeast to the food processor. Process until everything is combined.

Add all the herbs and salt to the food processor. Add the flax mixture and ⅓ cup of breadcrumbs to the food processor, and process until well combined.

Spread the remaining ¼ cup of breadcrumbs on a plate. Using a spoon, scoop up some of the tempeh mix and roll it into a ball, about the size of a golf ball. Roll the tempeh meatball in the bread crumbs so that it's completely covered and set aside on a plate. Continue making meatballs until you use up all the tempeh mix.

Heat oil in a large skillet over medium-high heat. Add the tempeh meatballs and fry. Depending on the size of your skillet, you may need to fry them in batches. Make sure the meatballs brown on all sides. When they are browned, transfer the meatballs to a paper towel–lined plate.

Gently add the tempeh meatballs to the simmering marinara sauce. Let them cook about 10 minutes until they are heated through.

MEATY CHICKPEA MEATLOAF

This loaf is so packed with protein you'll feel your abs form as you eat it. Perfect as an entrée or on a sandwich or sub as leftovers.

Ingredients for meatloaf:

2 14-ounce cans or 3⅓ cups cooked chickpeas, drained and rinsed

1 onion, diced

2 celery stalks, chopped

2 carrots, diced

2 garlic cloves, minced

2 cups gluten-free panko breadcrumbs

½ cup unsweetened non-dairy milk

3 tablespoons vegan Worcestershire sauce

2 tablespoons wheat-free tamari

2 tablespoons olive oil, plus extra to grease

2 tablespoons ground flax seeds

2 tablespoon tomato paste

1 teaspoon smoked paprika

¼ teaspoon black pepper

Ingredients for glaze:

⅓ cup ketchup

⅓ cup wheat-free tamari

Preheat oven to 375°F. Working in batches if needed, place all meatloaf ingredients into a food processor and pulse until chickpeas are broken up and ingredients are well mixed, stopping to scrape down sides of the food processor as needed. Do not overblend. If working in batches, transfer each batch to a large mixing bowl when complete and then mix by hand. If you're using an immersion blender, you may be able to do this all at once.

Press mixture into a lightly greased loaf pan and bake 30 minutes.

While meatloaf bakes, stir glaze ingredients together in a small bowl. Remove loaf from oven after 30 minutes and spoon glaze over top of loaf. Bake for another 20–25 minutes. Remove from oven and allow to cool for at least 10 minutes before slicing. Serve with french fries and ketchup.

VEGAN RANCH DRESSING

You know you're going to want to dip. Whether it's wings or french fries, this super-simple vegan ranch dressing tastes exactly like its dairy counterpart, since it consists of the same exact ingredients. Veganized, of course.

Ingredients:

1 cup vegan mayonnaise (Just Mayo)

½ teaspoon onion powder

½ teaspoon garlic powder

¼ teaspoon black pepper

2 tablespoons fresh parsley, chopped

½ cup unsweetened nondairy milk

Whisk all ingredients together and chill before serving. Add a little more milk if you need to thin the dressing for pouring or keep it thick for dipping.

CHEESY FUNDIDO DIP

Our local Tex-Mex restaurant makes an amazing fundido, a melted cheese you spoon onto warmed tortillas, which you then fold and place into your fundido-eating hole. Of course, that's not vegan. This is, and it's just as good. You can either use store-bought soy chorizo (I recommend Trader Joe's brand) or use the Chorizoats recipe in this book (page 222). Either way, this bowl of melted cheesy goodness is sure to please.

Ingredients:

1 cup unsweetened nondairy milk

1 package shredded vegan
   cheddar cheese

¼ cup nutritional yeast

2 tablespoons chili powder

1 package soy chorizo
   (or 2 cups Chorizoats on page
   222)

Soft corn tortillas

In a small pan, heat the milk over medium to low heat, adding the cheese a quarter cup at a time, stirring constantly. Keep adding cheese until it's all melted. Stir in the nutritional yeast and chili powder.

Transfer to large bowl and fold in the soy chorizo. Warm the corn tortillas for 20 minutes on low in an oven.

Serve individual small bowls of the fundido with a few warmed tortillas or chips.

NACHOS VEGANO

There's nothing like a huge plate of nachos piled high to center around a stand-up party. These are so satisfying and easy to make, you'll run the risk of making them too often. And since they're vegan, they're also healthy for you! Yeah . . . right.

Ingredients:

1 avocado
2 tablespoons garlic powder
1 lime, juiced
Pinch sea salt
Bag organic tortilla chips
1 16-ounce can of black beans

Bag shredded vegan cheddar cheese
2 fresh jalapeños, sliced
1 red onion, sliced
1 jar of your favorite hot salsa
Cilantro, chopped
Vegan sour cream, to serve

To make ½ cup of guacamole, remove the meat from the avocado and mash it with the back of a fork (never make guacamole in a food processor; it turns into green foam). Add garlic powder, juice from one lime, and a pinch of sea salt.

Arrange your tortilla chips on a large lightly greased cookie sheet and add the beans and cheese. Bake in a 400°F oven for 15 minutes until the cheese starts to melt (inasmuch as vegan cheese melts).

Remove from oven and transfer onto a large serving platter. Top with the jalapeños and red onion and drizzle on some salsa (save the rest of dipping). Top with cilantro, dip into the guacamole, and serve with vegan sour cream—because everything should be served with vegan sour cream.

CHICK'N SPIEDIE SANDWICH

My old Binghamton favorite, veganized (see page 8 to find out what a spiedie sandwich is). The tricky part of this recipe is that it requires one ingredient that's tough to find: at some Asian markets, the freezer section will contain a sausage-sized loaf of soy product that's usually labeled "vegan chicken." Other commercially available vegan chicken will work with this recipe, but that thicker loaf allows for nice 1 ½-inch cubes to be cut in the true Spiedie tradition. If you can't find this soy log, use Beyond Meat chicken strips since they hold up well on skewers. Did I mention you'll need skewers?

Ingredients for Spiedie sauce (which is also commercially available):

⅓ cup olive oil

¼ cup lemon juice

¼ cup white vinegar

2 garlic cloves (finely chopped or pressed)

1 tablespoon dried parsley

1 tablespoon dried basil

½ teaspoon dried oregano

½ teaspoon garlic salt

½ teaspoon salt

1 9-ounce packet vegan chicken product, cubed

Thin-sliced Italian bread

12 skewers (we use metal, but wood works, too; just soak ahead of time)

Spiedie sauce is essentially a vinaigrette. This is the original recipe from Lupo's, the home of the Spiedie sandwich. Whisk all of the ingredients for Spiedie sauce together.

Cut your chicken into 1- to 1½-inch cubes and marinade in a bath of Spiedie sauce in an airtight container. Leave overnight in the refrigerator.

The next day, skewer them up and slap on the grill, 5 minutes on each side. Place the chicken, skewer and all, onto a slice of bread and slide them off, folding the bread over the Spiedie meat. Consume.

NOTE: You can also use frozen tofu (defrosted, of course) for this recipe.

MAC 'N' CHEESE

I had to include a vegan macaroni and cheese recipe since we make this all the time. By adding nutritional yeast to this, you can get away with using almost any vegan cheese block (shredded) or a bag of shredded cheddar. Experiment until you find your favorite. Use elbow macaroni for the most authentic looking result or penne if you want it to look fancier.

Ingredients:

1 bag dried macaroni/pasta

2 cups unsweetened nondairy milk

1 bag shredded vegan cheddar cheese

½ cup vegan cream cheese (Tofutti is our favorite)

½ cup nutritional yeast

2 tablespoons turmeric

Pinch salt

¼ cup gluten-free/vegan panko-style bread crumbs (optional)

Prepare the macaroni according to the directions on the packet. Strain and set aside.

In a large pot, bring the milk up to a simmer and slowly add the vegan cheese until it has all been incorporated (stirring constantly, about 5 minutes). Stir in the cream cheese, nutritional yeast, turmeric, and salt.

Lower heat to low and stir in the macaroni until coated completely. You can serve as is or transfer to a large baking dish, top with breadcrumbs, and bake for 30 minutes in a 400°F oven until bread crumbs become crunchy.

JUMPER POTATOES

I've traveled to London once or twice and fell in love with their language. It's so much like American English, with a few notable exceptions: *exit* is *way out*, *suspenders* are *braces*, and *potato skins* are *jacket potatoes*. I love the image of a potato wearing a jacket, which, by the way, the British call *jumpers*, so I've decided to call my vegan potato skins "Jumper Potatoes" as a tribute to all my vegan mates across the pond. Here's to you, Michael Bosanko.

Ingredients:

5–6 medium-large russet potatoes
3 tablespoons oil, plus extra to rub
   on potatoes
½ teaspoon smoked paprika
¼ teaspoon garlic powder
¼ teaspoon salt
¼ teaspoon pepper

½ cup vegan cheddar cheese,
   grated
2 tablespoons vegan bacon bits,
   chopped (rice paper bacon
   recipe is on page 218)
6 green onions, thinly sliced, plus
   extra to garnish
Vegan sour cream

Preheat oven to 400°F. Poke a bunch of holes all over your potatoes with a fork so they don't explode, then treat them to a rubdown with a little olive oil. Toss the potatoes in the oven and bake for 40 minutes, or until you can easily stab them with a fork.

Remove from oven and slice potatoes in half lengthwise, being careful not to tear the skins. Raise oven temperature to 450°F and get ready to rumble.

With a spoon, scoop out the centers of the potatoes, leaving about ¼ inch or less of potato around the edges. Be careful not to puncture the skin while disemboweling them.

In a small bowl, stir together oil and spices. With a basting brush, coat the outer skins of the potatoes with oil mixture. In another bowl, toss vegan cheese with vegan bacon bits and a handful of thinly sliced green onions.

Top the potato skins with the cheese mixture and put them on an ungreased baking sheet. Bake for 8–10 minutes, and then stick 'em in the broiler for another 30 seconds, or until cheese is melted and skins are as crisp as you want them. Top each one with a dollop of vegan sour cream and plenty of green onions. Serve hot.

TOFU SCRAMBLE

We make this a few times a week. Sometimes, we wrap the scramble and some cheese up in a brown rice wrap and heat in a pan until the cheese is melty. You can take this basic tofu scramble and serve with hash browns, toast, and fresh fruit for an incredibly tasty and protein-packed start to your day. Or have breakfast for dinner. This very easy recipe is made easier if you can find organic chopped peppers and onions in your grocer's frozen food section.

Ingredients:

Olive oil, for sautéing
½ cup onions chopped
1 cup multicolored peppers
1 jalapeño pepper, chopped (optional)
1 cup chopped broccoli florets
1 brick organic firm tofu
⅓ cup nutritional yeast

1 tablespoon turmeric
1 teaspoon kala namak salt (gives it an authentic "eggy" taste)
Parsley, chopped (optional, to taste)
Salt, to taste
Pepper, to taste
Vegan mayo (optional)

Heat your nonstick frying pan to medium heat and add a little olive oil. Stir in the chopped onion and peppers (jalapeño is optional) and sauté for 10 minute until tender. Add the broccoli and cook for an additional 2–3 minutes.

Squeeze any excess water from the tofu brick over the sink and hand-crumble directly into the frying pan, breaking the tofu apart to the consistency of scrambled eggs. Stir tofu into the vegetables and add the nutritional yeast, turmeric, kala namak, and chopped parsley.

Continue to cook over medium heat until some edges of tofu begin to crisp (another 10 minutes). Salt and pepper to taste. To make this scramble come alive, stir in a tablespoon of vegan mayo (optional) at the end for added fat and creaminess.

BANANA HAMMOCK SHAKES
GIVE ME THE SHAKES

Three ingredients meet blender. We make variations of these all the time for the kids. So simple and delicious, and no dairy ice cream needed. Start with the basic recipe and then add more tasty ingredients (optional).

Basic ingredients:
2 frozen ripe bananas (peel and cut into pieces before freezing)
2 cups nondairy milk (sweetened/vanilla)
1 tablespoon vanilla extract

Put all three ingredients into the blender and let it rip. Within 3 minutes on high speed, you'll have a delicious, nutritious vanilla shake.

Want to really make it memorable? Try these tasty variations!

The Elvis Presley
Throw in a quarter cup of peanut butter and a handful of vegan dark chocolate chips (optional) during the last minute of blending.

The Banana Hammock
Toss in a quarter cup of shredded coconut and serve with a slice of pineapple, mon.

Wake Me Up Before You Go Go
Toss in a half cup of strong, black, cold coffee.

The US Mint
Add 2 tablespoons of peppermint extract (sold wherever baking supplies are sold) and a handful of vegan dark chocolate chips (optional) during the last minute of blending.

Chocolate Rain

Ahlaska brand makes an amazing vegan organic chocolate syrup that you can add. Oddly enough, Hershey's brand of chocolate syrup is also vegan (but loaded with other junk you don't want).

Strawberry Feels Forever

It's always great having frozen fruits and vegetables on hand, and here's one more reason why. Add ½ cup of frozen strawberries to your shake and delight in how much it reminds you of strawberry Nesquik.

Substitutions in the Kitchen

Whether you're baking a cake or making a vegan shepherd's pie, you're going to discover that there is a replacement for every ingredient that is vegan. From simply replacing eggs with applesauce or milk with almond milk, nearly every recipe (or boxed cake mix) can be veganized. For all recipes that call for milk, simply replace with an equal amount of your favorite nondairy milk. Same for butter. Eggs are a little trickier but shouldn't slow you down in the least. While you can use off-the-shelf egg substitutes, there are also easy, tasty, and less expensive options already in your kitchen.

For sweeter recipes (cakes/cupcakes, etc) simply use organic apple sauce or a mashed ripe banana (¼ cup = 1 egg), and for savory recipes refer to this egg-cellent chart:

Ingredient	+ Water	Equals
1 tablespoon ground flax seed	3 tablespoons	1 egg
1 tablespoon chia seeds	⅓ cup	1 egg
1 tablespoon soy protein	3 tablespoons	1 egg
1 tablespoon agar agar	1 tablespoon	1 egg

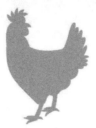

EPILOGUE

It takes nothing away from a human to be kind to an animal.
—Joaquin Phoenix

I've said it before, and I'll say it again: the way I was eating for the first half of my life was not going to make the second half go well. Meat, dairy, and eggs were killing me, and they're slowly killing you (if you've decided to still eat them after reading this book). There will be warning labels on these products one day, and then we vegans can say, "We told you so."

At forty-five, the true "middle age," you can look back and reflect on all the fun you had as a kid. The decisive, and still wild, twenties and the settling-down thirties. You've reached a milestone at forty, and then you turn that corner toward a half decade. Buckle up. It's the point in your life where wrinkles start appearing, spots on your skin come from out of nowhere, your hair starts to turn grey and grow in strange places or recede altogether, and your vision worsens. It's like cruel puberty.

It's also the age where staying fit becomes much more challenging. Keeping the pounds off and the belt in the same notch is more challenging still. Your metabolism changes; it's a fact of life. If you are one of the lucky few who doesn't have to worry about this, great, but for the rest of us, changes need to take place, and it's never too late for them to happen.

Veganism is not a sacrifice. It is a joy.
—Gary L. Francione

Going vegan is not easy for anyone. Especially for older people who have eaten as omnivores their entire lives. But it can be done, and the rewards far outweigh the downsides. From a dietary perspective, it is an ideal time to take your health into your own hands (prying it from big meat and pharmaceutical industries), controlling what goes into your body as fuel, and truly feeling the health benefits. When cancer can be turned off and on by introducing or taking away dairy, or cured by eating strawberries as shown through the research compiled by Dr. Greger and NutritionFacts.org, I'm shocked when I see people still subscribing to the old way of thinking when it comes to food and their health.

Shortly after you've truly begun eating a vegan diet, you realize you are losing weight while you're eating more. You realize that vegan food is adventurous and delicious. You'll suddenly make "the connection." Pigs are not bacon. Cows are not steaks. And chickens are not . . . well, actually, they'll still be chickens. The whole thing starts to make sense. You are living a healthy and compassionate second half of your life. You can look at every meal and know that it is nourishing your body and your soul.

You'll also know you're helping the planet.

It's at this point that you'll welcome the ripe age of fifty. Instead of "pushing it," know that when it comes to the importance of being vegan, you really shouldn't be skeptical.

Every living creature has the right to live ethically.
—*Dirk Verbeuren*

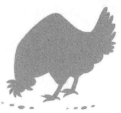

ACKNOWLEDGMENTS

Let us be grateful to the people who make us happy;
they are the charming gardeners who make our souls blossom.
—Marcel Proust

L eonardo Da Vinci said, "The time will come when men such as I will look upon the murder of animals as they now look upon the murder of men." While I hope for this in my lifetime, I feel it may only happen a few generations after I am gone. So, it's up to my kids' kids, which is one of the many reasons why we are raising them vegan. One day, everyone's eyes will be opened to veganism, and we will live in a more peaceful coexistence with one another: humans and animals together.

There are so many amazing people I've met along my own journey to veganism who have somehow, in their own ways, made this book possible. I am so proud to be a member of the vegan community and admire all the hard work you all do every day for the animals.

To my mom, who raised the three of us, along with Nana and George, for the absolute best childhood anyone could ever ask for. We didn't have money, but we never felt like we needed it. We had love. And dinner together every night. As a matter of fact, we were so poor growing up that we had to wear synthetic rubber sneakers that looked like leather sneakers. I used to draw the Adidas logo on the back with a Sharpie marker so no one would know. Little did I know then that, one day, I would actually be looking for these vegan sneakers on purpose.

To Jen for finding me, believing in me, and turning my life around. You mean more to me than you could ever imagine and have opened my eyes to so much. You also somehow talked me into having more babies, and for that I am forever grateful. I never knew how off-track I was until I met you. You took the raw material and helped form the man I am today—and for that I love you.

To my babies, the two little ones and the one big one (my little monkey). You are my reason for being and succeeding. I want you to learn from my life, mistakes and all. I hope you'll forever look at me the way you look at me today. I'm looking to you to change the world. No pressure.

To Meena, for being that precocious ten-year-old and insisting we try veganism. It's because of you that I am where I am today and that I can share my story with so many other potential vegans.

I have long dreamt of writing a book, and the daunting task of my weekly word count updates toward reaching my eighty-one-thousand-long word count seemed impossible at times. Did I have enough to say? Could I string together that many words to write something readable? In your hands is the result of this effort, and I hope you've enjoyed it.

I couldn't thank Skyhorse Publishing and my editor, Kim Lim, enough for the opportunity.

And thank you to others who have contributed something meaningful to my life or this book:

Mark Anbinder

Ed Baptist

David Benzaquen

Rob Bigwood

Michael Bosanko

Nelson Campbell

T. Colin Campbell

Dr. Tom Campbell

Sherry Colb

John Corry

Christine Day

Michael Dorf

Robin Everson

Cindy Ford

Lewis Freedman

Daisy Fuentes

Steve Glover

David Hall

Amie Hamlin

Alex Hershaft

Matthew Hranek

Steve Jenks

Hadley Johnson

Kathleen Keene

Steffi Koroka
Benji Kurtz
Kristin Lajeunesse
Gillian Lindstrom
Joann Lindstrom
Peg Lindstrom
Lexi Love
Sean Lunny
Jen Majka
Perri Mandelbaum
Kayle Martin
Richard Marx
Sly Mata
Tracye McQuirter
Jenny Miller
Matthew Modine
Justin Moore-Brown
Victoria Moran

Colleen Patrick-Goudreau
Brian Patton
Ashlee Piper
Laura Prevost
Ruby Roth
Doug Russell
Alessandra Savoia
Miyoko Schinner
Skyhorse Publishing
Michael Suchman
Priscilla Timberlake
Kristy Turner
Chris VanDruff
My vegan babies
Samantha Waldo
Brian Wendel
Jason Wrobel

Contributors: Cindy Ford (SillyLittleVegan.com), Christine Day (ANewDayVegan.com), Sherry Colb (*Mind If I Order the Cheeseburger?*), Michael Dorf (*Beating Hearts: Abortion and Animal Rights (Critical Perspectives on Animals: Theory, Culture, Science, and Law)*), and Michael Suchman (*VeganMos*).

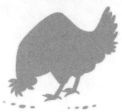

NOTES

Pg. ix. Ruby Roth, *That's Why We Don't Eat Animals: A Book About Vegans, Vegetarians, and All Living Things* (North Atlantic Books, 2009).

Pg. xiii. Sherry Colb, *Mind If I Order the Cheeseburger?: And Other Questions People Ask Vegans* (Lantern Books, 2013).

Pg. xiii. T. Colin Campbell, *The China Study* (BenBella Books, 2006).

Pg. 1. Albert Einstein, letter to Hans Muehsam, March 30, 1954.

Pg. 13. "Diets high in meat, eggs and dairy could be as harmful to health as smoking," *The Guardian*, March 5, 2014. https://www.theguardian.com/science/2014/mar/04/animal-protein-diets-smoking-meat-eggs-dairy.

Pg. 19. "Researchers Find New Link Between Red Meat and Heart Disease (Video)," *Cleveland Clinic*, November 11, 2014. https://health.clevelandclinic.org/2014/11/researchers-find-new-link-between-red-meat-and-heart-disease-video/.

Pg. 27. Jeremy Bentham, *An Introduction to the Principles of Morals and Legislation*, 1789.

Pg. 32. T. F. Hodge, *From Within I Rise: Spiritual Triumph over Death and Conscious Encounters with "The Divine Presence"* (PublishAmerica, 2009).

Pg. 44. Colleen Patrick-Goudreau, *The 30-Day Vegan Challenge* (Ballantine Books, 2011).

Pg. 51. Albert Einstein, letter to Hans Muehsam, March 30, 1954.

Pg. 55. Peter M. Senge, *The Fifth Discipline: The Art & Practice of the Learning Organization* (Doubleday, 2006).

Pg. 56. Moby, *The End of Everything* essay, Elektra, 1996.

Pg. 69. Sarah Taylor, *Vegetarian to Vegan* (The Vegan Next Door, 2013).

Pg. 78. Carl Sagan, *The Varieties of Scientific Experience: A Personal View of the Search for God* (Penguin Books, 2007).

Pg. 84. Michael Klaper, qtd. in David Robinson Simon, *Meatonomics* (Conari Press, 2013).

Pg. 89. Paul Simon, qtd. in Jon Landau, "Paul Simon: The Rolling Stone Interview," *Rolling Stone*, July 20, 1972.

Pg. 98. Dolly Parton, qtd. in Bryan Miller, "AT LUNCH WITH: Dolly Parton; For 'Friendly Country Clod,' A Day for Charming the City," *New York Times*, April 29, 1992.

Pg. 100. John McDougall, *The Starch Solution: Eat the Foods You Love, Regain Your Health, and Lose the Weight for Good!* (Rodale Books, 2013).

Pg. 101. Chef AJ, *Unprocessed: How to Achieve Vibrant Health and Your Ideal Weight* (CreateSpace Publishing, 2011).

Pg. 103. Coldplay, "The Scientist," by Chris Martin, in *A Rush of Blood to the Head*, Capitol, 2002.

Pg. 111. Mark Bittman, *VB6: Eat Vegan Before 6:00 to Lose Weight and Restore Your Health . . . For Good* (Clarkson Potter, 2013).

Pg. 116. Stephen King, "Everything You Need to Know About Writing Successfully—in Ten Minutes," in Sylvia K. Burack (Ed.) *The Writer's Handbook* (Writer, Inc., 1988): 3–9.

Pg. 131. Eric Carle, *The Very Hungry Caterpillar* (Philomel Books, 1994).

Pg. 131. Lois Ehlert, *Eating the Alphabet* (HMH Books for Young Readers, 1996).

Pg. 132. Ruby Roth, *Vegan Is Love: Having Heart and Taking Action* (North Atlantic Books, 2012).

Pg. 132. Ruby Roth, *The Help Yourself Cookbook for Kids* (Andrews McMeel Publishing, 2016).

Pg. 138. César Chávez, accepting a Lifetime Achievement Award from In Defense of Animals (June 14, 1992).

Pg. 154. Caldwell Esselstyn, Jr., *Prevent and Reverse Heart Disease: The Revolutionary, Scientifically Proven, Nutrition-Based Cure* (Avery, 2008).

Pg. 157. Peter Singer, *Animal Liberation: The Definitive Classic of the Animal Movement* (Harper Perennial Modern Classics, 2009).

Pg. 165. Chris Hedges, "I've Gone Vegan to Help Try to Save the Planet," *Alternet.org*, November 10, 2014. http://www.alternet.org/environment/chris-hedges-ive-gone-vegan-help-try-save-planet.

Pg. 171. Colleen Patrick-Goudreau, *The Joy of Vegan Baking: The Compassionate Cooks' Traditional Treats and Sinful Sweets* (Fair Winds Press, 2007).

Pg. 179. Erma Bombeck, *Forever, Erma: Best-Loved Writing from America's Favorite Humorist* (Andrews McMeel Publishing, 1996).

Pg. 181. Dave Barry, qtd. in *Snark! The Herald Angels Sing: Sarcasm, Bitterness, and the Holiday Season* by Lawrence Dorfman (Skyhorse Publishing, 2011).

Pg. 190. Howard Schultz, qtd. in Carmine Gallo, "What Starbucks CEO Howard Schultz Taught Me about Communication and Success," *Forbes*, December 19, 2013.

Pg. 192. Morrissey, *Autobiography* (Penguin Classics, 2014).

Pg. 199. Jiminy Cricket, *Pinocchio* (Walt Disney Pictures, 1940).

Pg. 202. Lindsay Nixon, *The Happy Herbivore Cookbook* (BenBella Books, 2011).

Pg. 209. Erykah Badu, qtd. in "Erykah Badu," *VegNews*, October 6, 2008.